TESTIMONIALS

A rare and powerful synthesis of science and spirit. Sarah reveals the spine as a living intelligence—one that reshapes how you understand your body, your mind, and your life.

David The Medium

A beautiful way to see our humanness. It feels like coming home to your body and yourself.

Dr Anthea Todd

In a world that is constantly trying to define, control, and normalize the human body, Sarah has chosen to do something very different. She has chosen to listen to it.

Through Spinal Energetics, she is revealing something most people have forgotten: that the body is an intelligent and responsive structure that is deeply connected to an energetic field that guides everything beneath the surface.

What makes her work powerful is that she allows the body to express, move and release without forcing it into a predetermined shape. In doing so, she gives people permission to witness a deeper truth—that healing emerges from within when the right conditions are created.

She is showing that what has been labeled as unusual, emotional, or even uncomfortable is often the body reorganizing itself in real time.

That takes clarity. That takes trust. And it takes courage.

This book is an invitation for people to reconnect with their own body, to trust it, and to experience what becomes possible when they do.

Garry Lineham – Human Garage

YOUR SPINE HOLDS THE ANSWER

YOUR SPINE HOLDS THE ANSWER

THE STORY YOU'VE BEEN CARRYING

DR SARAH JANE PERRI

First published in 2026 by Dean Publishing
PO Box 119
Mt. Macedon, Victoria, 3441
Australia
deanpublishing.com

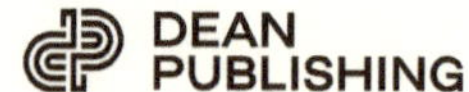

Cataloguing-in-Publication Data
National Library of Australia
Title: Your Spine Holds the Answer—The Story You've Been Carrying
ISBN: 978-1-764372-32-9
Category: Health/chiropractic

The views and opinions expressed in this book are those of the author and do not necessarily reflect the official policy or position of any other agency, publisher, organization, employer, medical body, psychological body, or company. Assumptions made in the analysis are not reflective of the position of any entity other than the author(s) – and, these views are always subject to change, revision, and rethinking at any time.

The author, publisher or organisations are not to be held responsible for misuse, reuse, recycled and cited and/or uncited copies of content within this book by others.

The information in this book is for educational and informational purposes only and is not intended as medical advice, diagnosis, or treatment. While Spinal Energetics and the concepts presented may support wellbeing, they are not a substitute for professional medical care.

Readers are encouraged to consult with a qualified healthcare provider regarding any medical condition or health concerns. The author and publisher disclaim any liability arising directly or indirectly from the use or application of the information contained in this book.

These words are dedicated to my mother, Nella. Thank you for teaching me the considerable gift of the "small" things and for cultivating a love that gave me the freedom to discover my legitimate self in the world of falsehoods and expectations. There is an unceasing and profound ache within my heart that by no means will ever truly be reconciled. But that deep dejection is all of my entirety's honour. I hold an immense magnitude of appreciation for allowing your pain to become my grace and fortitude in this lifetime.

To Dr. Carli Axford, thank you for inspiring me to study chiropractic. Life without this would be life without air. Thank you for your support and for showing me what is possible. I have no doubt that our paths crossing was kismet—what a beautiful reminder of the things that are meant to be.

CONTENTS

PART TWO: THE LANGUAGE OF THE SPINE

PART THREE: THE STORY YOU'RE CARRYING

PRELUDE

Not everything that shaped me is visible.
But it's all here: in the work I do, the ways
I love and the spaces I create.
This is who I am.

Like many, grief has shaped me. It morphed its way into my bones and marinated itself in my flesh. Five miscarriages left untold stories behind. Tales of broken dreams and lifeless promises.

A DQ alpha gene was the culprit. My ex-husband and I happened to be a rare immune match, meaning both of us carry the same gene. My body couldn't tell the difference between an embryo and a threat. Albeit, our babies didn't grow.

Although I haven't lost the possibility of motherhood, I did lose the future I was building at that time. That dream. That family. Those babies. Those possibilities.

This realization didn't land softly—it pummeled me with loss, stigma and loneliness.

IVF followed and I created embryos in hope. But life had other plans.

We were then approved for surrogacy; a system loaded with red tape, expenses, delays, and legal barriers. My sister-in-law offered to carry our baby, but received brutal news when she was diagnosed with an eye tumor.

I had to let go of that hope. Again and again. I also had to let go of my marriage.

At the same time, the mother I once knew was lost too, but not to death. She quickly developed ADEM, a rare inflammatory brain disease. Within days of getting the first headache, she was in a coma and brain damaged. Her frontal lobe was massacred from lesions invading both her brain and spine. From one week to the next, we had reversed roles. The mother who raised me was suddenly childlike. I became her carer while miscarrying my fourth pregnancy.

Two mothers lost in one season.

She remembers the past, but not the present. A smart and beautiful woman who was once so proud lost the dignity she'd carried her whole life. She lost her ability to mother, to function, to create, and to live well.

We were pushed out of hospitals and rehab too soon. I was told to take her home but received minimal support. Navigating aged care, disability systems, and home care exhausted me. I white-knuckled my way through the pain, all while grieving and struggling.

I was swept into a shitstorm with no compass. Caregivers often are. You're suddenly swimming in deep waters and expected to become a nurse, advocate, social worker and emotional rock overnight.

To me, this wasn't just a crisis—it was a rupture of trust in a system meant to support us. My initiation into being a carer came with a confronting and sobering truth: we were invisible in a system not built to hold us.

Six years on and it's not much easier. Mum has been living in aged care full-time since she was 69. I miss the woman she was, but I am equally proud of the woman she is.

I guess life shapes us in ways we don't see coming. Our stories live inside of us. The good, the glorious, the ugly, the shameful, the untold.

One thing I know for sure is that our bodies hold our stories. They are the backbone of our lives. The vessel in which we collect and keep our inner narratives.

Our bodies know first. But they are very good at keeping scars and secrets in the vault of our flesh, bone and blood.

This book reveals how we can release the stories that load us but keep the lessons they blessed us with. How we can recognize what holds us back and what moves us forward. How we can ignite our best selves and heal our wounds. How we can liberate ourselves physically and metaphysically and honor the stories that shaped us.

Just as a book's spine holds the story inside, our spines hold the archives of our stories—spoken and unspoken, lived and unlived. They carry burdens and lovingly bend and flex to all resistance. But this does not mean they don't carry a toll. The stories that live inside of us shape us in mysterious ways. We become the stories we carry. Our spines are the library system of us.

And I believe the most radical act of care is creating beauty where pain has lived.

That's what this book is about. Your spine is your salvation.

Let me show you how.

INTRODUCTION

I get a little envious when I see babies and kids going to the chiropractor because I was 22 when I first found chiropractic. I was finishing my psychology degree and working as a fashion buyer, which is someone who selects and purchases clothes and accessories for retailers to stock. Although I love all things design, fashion and art, being a fashion buyer had no spiritual inspiration for me. I didn't feel like I was being of service in a meaningful way. I was not changing the world like my soul longed to.

I knew there was something else for me, I just didn't know what it was. I investigated naturopathy and similar holistic fields. I didn't want to be a conventional doctor and despite my degree, I didn't want to be a conventional psychologist either.

There was a mismatch between me and the career trajectory I was searching for. So in my quest for alignment, I typed the word "meaningful" into a job search engine. Only one job popped up. It was a chiropractic position for Dr. Carli Axford, the creator of Spinal Flow. I didn't know a lot about chiropractic, but figured it was similar to physiotherapy. How naive I was.

I applied and Dr. Carli rang me for an interview. On the phone, I quickly blurted out that I didn't have any experience in chiropractic but that I'd typed the word "meaningful" into a job search engine.

"It's meant to be," she said.

The moment I walked into the clinic, I felt a sense of home. Something familiar stirred within me. Something innate. I scanned the room. They stocked the same books that I read, and a peaceful Buddha statue was nestled on the reception desk. Everyone was walking around barefoot. Peace hummed through my body and nestled into my cells.

During the interview, I somehow talked Dr. Carli into giving me the job. I was a chiropractic assistant, and although I didn't work with clients, I managed all the comings and goings and saw the inner framework of running a clinic. I also got to see the "before" and "after" of chiropractic work. I was colliding with destiny and something within me knew it.

Over time in the clinic, I noticed that people were coming in for back, neck or knee pain but left with so much more. That got me thinking. People came in for pain management but also made noticeable shifts emotionally, mentally or spiritually. Clients often reported positive changes in their relationships or careers and linked it to the treatment they received. I started to notice patterns of connections and saw old patterns melt away through spinal work.

I'd never seen that before and it had me intrigued.

I must admit, I haven't seen that in many traditional chiropractic clinics so it's not common. I sensed its importance but didn't yet understand "the source" of such deep transformation. Of course it involved the spine and the nervous system, but it wasn't as simple or as specific as only pain relief.

I worked with other chiropractors at the same time and noticed people did get pain relief, but they didn't see the same kind of deep change in other areas of their life. I began to reflect on what Carli did differently. It became evident that she worked on the spine, the sacrum, and the neck in a tonal way. She listened to the body's energetic wave patterns and removed the blockages in order to get spinal flow.

I knew there was something special to pay attention to, yet I was still asking myself career defining questions. I became a holistic counselor as that seemed more fitting with my psychology degree. I also investigated kinesiology and completed a Reiki course because I really didn't want to go back and study for another five years to become a chiropractor. And when I say really, I mean really, really didn't want to go back because I had just completed four years of study.

Then one day Carli came in and said, "I'm moving to Bali. I'm changing my life and I'm getting rid of the clinic." I was left reeling, as I had a half plan to take over the clinic. I didn't want to go to Bali with her, as I had just gotten engaged, so I was left floundering.

I tried working as a practice manager at other clinics, but I wasn't fulfilled because I just wanted to be the chiropractor. I wanted to be the person helping, the conduit for relieving suffering and opening new possibilities.

Despite my resistance to more study, I ended up applying to university again and just accepted that it would take five more years of investment to get where I wanted to be.

And that's how the spine and I had a date with destiny. I released my resistance to study and said yes to the bigger plan that God had waiting for me.

Spine 101

The only thing I knew about the spine before my chiro degree was spinal subluxation. The simple theory that the spine is misaligned and interferes in the natural communication between the mind and body. The misalignment impacts the central nervous system and reduces the ability to function well. The spine gets manipulated back into alignment and symptoms decrease. Voila.

But I noticed that some clients would go to their chiropractor three or four times a week in order to retrain the spine. And while they would initially see progress, they would ultimately plateau. I became curious about this and sensed there was a missing puzzle piece.

I suspected that doing the same adjustments over and over didn't make it novel for the body. I wondered if the brain could predict what was going to happen. Like going to the gym for the first time and lifting a five-kilogram weight. Initially, that weight may extend you and change the body, but six weeks later you need a different program. You can't just have the same workout and expect different results. The same happens in pharmacology, as the body builds up a resistance to certain medications, often higher doses or new medication is needed to achieve the same effects.

That type of traditional chiro treatment didn't fully resonate with me. Our bodies aren't machines, they are dynamic intelligent living systems that move, breathe and balance, so adjusting the same way repeatedly didn't align with the radical transformations I had seen in Dr. Carli's clinic. I was searching for the pearl in the oyster, the ultimate jewel for health and change.

The other aspect of traditional chiro that clashed with my own belief system was the idea: why am I forcing a change in the body, thinking I know better than this person's body knows?

I wondered if there was a deeper wisdom in my client's body that silently said, "I need to function this way." To first create the subluxation, something had signaled to the body, "You need to alter, you need to move."

So what signaled that? The innate intelligence.

The same wisdom that digests your food and beats your heart. The same wisdom that moves your blood and grows your hair and nails. The same wisdom that tells you whether you're on the right track or veering off.

I began to question Chiro 101. If as a chiropractor, I am trying to manipulate the subluxation every time, are people really getting the change their body wants them to have? Are we dealing with the root causation? And what if the body could correct misalignment on its own?

If the body shifted it there in the first place, that means it can unshift it. But I needed to understand why it did it in the first place. What caused the shift?

This began my exploration into energetics. I was on a mission to find the root causation—not just working on the physical body, but looking at whether there was a mental, emotional or spiritual reason for our bodies' misalignments.

I dared to ask myself puzzling and unconventional questions. Questions like:

- *Could this physical imbalance or dysregulation be a result of their:*
  - ~ *Psychology*
  - ~ *Trauma*
  - ~ *Karma*
  - ~ *Dharma*
  - ~ *Conditioning*
  - ~ *Emotional stress*
  - ~ *Environment*
  - ~ *Spiritual destiny*
  - ~ *Awakening*
  - ~ *Personal growth*
  - ~ *Neglect*
- *What if the root causation was in these energetic fields first, and then it presented physically?*
- *If it started in the field, then why are we working only with the physical aspect in an attempt to change the field?*

I took a deep dive into vast fields of energetic medicine. Eastern and Western medicine, quantum physics, trauma psychology, bodywork, breathwork, integrative medicine.

The more I looked, the more I found, the more I connected dots and cross-bridged fields. I noticed that some of the world's leading scientists had asked the same big questions.

For example, American theoretical physicist Dr. David Bohm described the universe as The Implicate Order, suggesting that the universe is not made of separate parts, but is an undivided whole. He says that we are living in fields of manifested and unmanifested order that connects mind, matter, and consciousness.

Applying this to our bodies suggests we are not just a bunch of isolated cells in a single body but that we are connected to universal fields of energy and intelligence. We are bathing in fields with energetic patterns.

Neuroscience and psychology have also explored such deep connections. Dr. Carl Jung also saw the mind and body as a unified, inseparable system. He believed the unconscious expresses itself through physical symptoms and bodily sensations. That our bodies signal symptoms to us when the psyche is out of balance. He stated, "For what is the body? The body is merely the visibility of the soul, the psyche; and the soul is the psychological experience of the body."[1]

Even Einstein concluded that the "Body and soul are not two different things, but only two different ways of perceiving the same thing."

The whirlpool of knowledge from various fields of science, psychology, and philosophy coincided with my experiences and what I had witnessed in clients who had had radical changes. The interconnected nature of science, spine and spirit fused together and epiphany after epiphany began to reveal something.

Finally the physical and the energetic danced as one. The measurable and the meaningful joined. The integration of both East and West: science and soul, biology and mystery.

Over time and with much research and examination, what was born among my curiosity and frustration was something groundbreaking. It took years and years to crystallize the foundations of Spinal Energetics: a modality I founded that works with the physical and metaphysical fields to achieve freedom and health.

This modality didn't spring from a textbook, but it came from a melting pot of things: study and curiosity, watching people's recovery or regression in clinical practices, suffering from personal grief, and holding pain in my body and psyche. I had lived in the gaps.

It also arose from the realization that physical interventions often hit a ceiling. I would see clients with textbook physical issues but they weren't responding to textbook treatments. Their X-rays were clean, yet their pain was debilitating.

It became undeniable that the variable wasn't the bone or the muscle; it was the emotional and energetic load the person was carrying. The spine wasn't just supporting their weight; it was supporting their unintegrated trauma and emotional reality.

Lydia's Case Study

Take Lydia as an example. Lydia came to our clinic with "unexplained" neck and shoulder pain. If I had simply treated her physical symptoms, she may have felt better for a day or two, but then her symptoms would have reoccurred. But I asked Lydia about other changes (outside of her physical pain) that she'd experienced recently.

She told me that she had lost her job and was feeling very anxious about money. Now, a life challenge like this doesn't just stay in the mental and emotional field. It bleeds into the body and nervous system. It can affect your identity, your relationships, your feelings of security and safety. For Lydia, her posture changed. Tension accumulated through her neck and jaw, and she felt she had the weight of the world on her shoulders (and she physically and psychically did have that weight on her).

Without doing blood tests, I knew her cortisol levels would have increased, her flight-or-fight response would have kicked in, and her parasympathetic system would have been dysregulated. All this tension and stress changed her physiology and ignited symptoms. It was a combination of both her seen and unseen loads, her tangible and intangible burdens, her inner pain and her physical pain.

Lydia's pain presented itself physically. It indicated a message to her. If I had only focused on physical symptoms and neglected other forms of pain (like a critical life change), then her relief would only penetrate to a physical relief. Then once she went home and contemplated her deeper stress, the physiology patterns would have returned.

Now although I couldn't give Lydia a new job, I could work in the energetic fields of her psychology and belief system and help her feel safe and supported in her new circumstance. I could help facilitate an energetic shift in her identity and her body would make the adjustment.

No parts of us should be neglected or ignored as all parts make you whole. With Lydia, ignoring her new life circumstance would have been ignoring one of the most critical things happening in her life at the time.

Her invisible burden was evident in her tension and shoulder and neck pain.

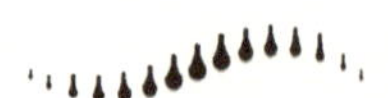

A lot of these deeper reasons are in the unconscious, not the conscious. You may not know consciously that you are holding them, but they appear in your body.

And that's the part I believe we're working with—the unconscious—which I believe resides in the spine and is the innate intelligence. Without working within those deeper parts of you, we're not working with all aspects of you. It's not merely a superficial thing or only a physical issue. It presents physically yes, but the source of it is often deeper.

This is what Spinal Energetics is founded on. It takes the whole person into account. It looks beyond the physical field and into the mental, emotional and spiritual fields to find the source of the pain or illness—communicating directly with the innate intelligence that told the body to display those symptoms in the first place.

It is here that we can finally listen to what the body is communicating to us through its physical manifestation. Our bodies are intelligent and they never have "random" symptoms. The physical manifestation is simply the innate intelligence trying to tell us to stop suppressing, stop burying our needs, and stop ignoring what we know we need to address.

"The only acceptable point of view appears to be the one that recognizes both sides of reality–the quantitative and the qualitative, the physical and the psychical–as compatible with each other, and can embrace them simultaneously."[2]

Wolfgang Ernst Pauli

The People in the Gaps

There is a place for conventional medicine, but what happens when the physical injuries and "mystery" illnesses like autoimmune diseases, gut issues and chronic fatigue don't appear on X-rays, MRI scans, or fail to indicate issues on blood tests?

Modern medicine is failing to treat these seemingly physical afflictions because when they investigate using the tools they have, nothing is detected. These are the people that fall between the gaps in the system. They are suffering but the medical tests insist "nothing is wrong." The tools don't provide an answer, and most conventional doctors aren't equipped with other methods on where else to find answers. If it doesn't fall into their medical check-a-box, it cannot be measured and therefore "does not exist" in medical terms. But it does exist! It just doesn't exist in the fixed parameters set by the healthcare system.

This is one of the many reasons why energetic work is increasingly important in the world we live in. Society is becoming increasingly more and more disconnected. Not only is our sense of community dissolving (and getting replaced by online imitations), but technology and our modern lifestyles have left us out of touch with our bodies, minds and souls. Research shows that in a world of "connectivity," we are experiencing an epidemic of disconnection from our bodies and emotions.[3]

So it's more important than ever that we become conscious of our whole selves and reconnect the lost or fragmented parts of ourselves.

Think of it like this, we cry when we're sad, we get a tight chest when we're anxious, and we shake when we are scared or nervous. The connection to our emotions and bodies is natural—what is unnatural is trying to suppress it and numb ourselves with television, social media, food, alcohol or drugs. We often have persistent pain but ignore it and swallow painkillers to cut off the connection. Or on a bigger level, we are often forced to live a life that isn't truly reflective of our true desires, so we suppress our dreams and console ourselves with meaningless tradeoffs.

But where do these emotions, pains and desires go when buried underneath the modern distractions? They linger in the body and become trapped underneath the busyness of our lives and apparent effectiveness of our coping mechanisms. They do not stay benign. Like a hose with a kink in it, the blockage eventually gets so strained, it has to release the pressure somewhere: the hose might burst or fray until it starts leaking out. Either way, what we suppress always finds a way back to the surface, whether we like it or not. *What we resist persists.*

When you think about it, it would be strange to go through trauma or stress and have it not show up in your body. Working energetically is not about eliminating everything either. It's about tuning into the body and the spine, listening to what it's communicating, and getting to the root cause of any issues. When working with the energetic field, people's bodies are moving and adjusting on their own to shift and rejig those tension patterns.

In many ways this premise isn't new. The Greek physician and father of medicine, Hippocrates, told us centuries ago that "When in sickness, look to the spine first."

This ancient wisdom coupled with today's maladies and culture is more necessary than ever. We have more connectivity but less connection. More health remedies but less health. More information but less transformation.

So, let's look to the spine first and see what we can find.

"When in sickness,
look to the spine first."

HIPPOCRATES

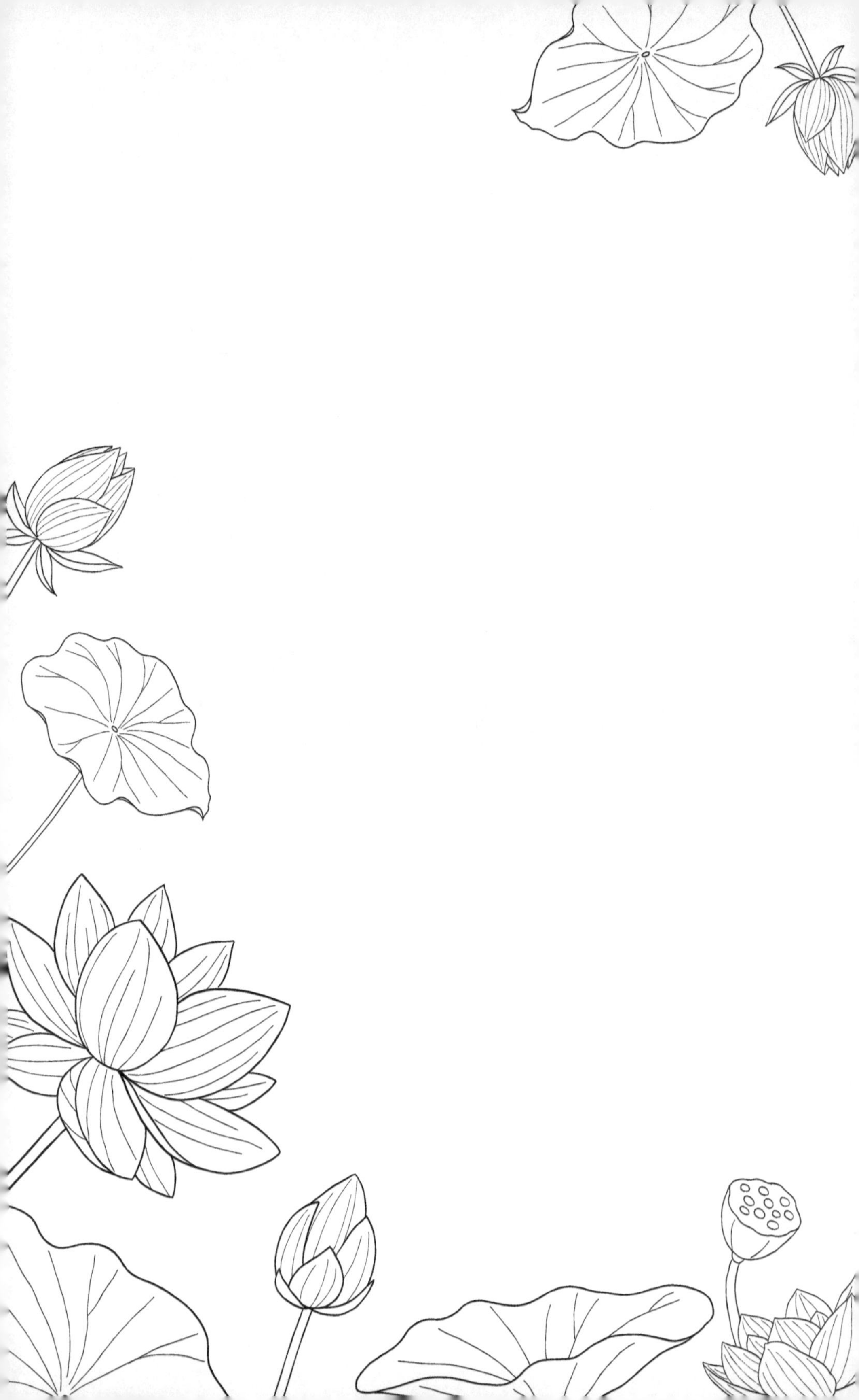

PART ONE

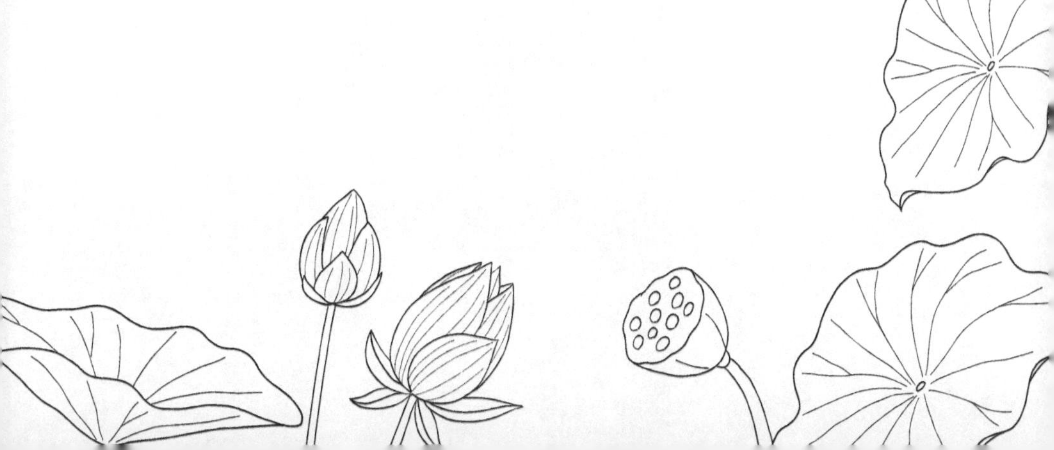

CHAPTER 1

The Silent Architect

Demystifying Innate Intelligence

Spinal Energetics is based on three main premises.

1. There is an innate intelligence within us that governs our health.
2. Our bodies are surrounded by energetic fields that reflect the workings of that intelligence.
3. Our bodies and minds are integrated systems that constantly influence one another.

To understand Spinal Energetics, it's important to ground the practice in established scientific principles and facts, along with ancient knowledge that has always been intuitively powerful.

For the Western mind, believing in what we cannot see is a tall order. We are a culture built on the tangible, the measurable, and the solid. We are taught from a young age that if you can't touch it, weigh it, or measure it, it likely doesn't exist. So if the term "innate intelligence" sounds too mystical or woo-woo for you, let's strip away the language and look at the biology.

At its core, innate intelligence is simply the silent operating system of life. It is the inherent wisdom that organizes matter into life.

You don't need to "believe" in it, because you are living it. It is the force that is beating your heart, digesting your breakfast, and replacing your skin cells right now, all without a single conscious command from you. If you had to consciously manage your thyroid levels or tell your kidneys how to filter toxins, you wouldn't survive past lunch.

Now, if you come from a medical background, you might rightly point out: "That isn't magic; that's the brain stem."

And you would be correct.

Biologically, the brain stem (specifically structures like the medulla oblongata) acts as the control center for your autonomic nervous system. It is the master switchboard that regulates your respiration, heart rate and blood pressure. It is the physical hardware that keeps the machine running.

But in Spinal Energetics, we ask: *What powers the hardware?*

Think of your body like a supercomputer. The brain stem is the CPU—the processor that executes the commands. But a processor cannot run without software, and it cannot run without electricity. Innate intelligence is that electricity. It is the signal running through the brain stem, the animating life force that tells the autonomic nervous system how to maintain homeostasis (balance) in a constantly changing environment.

The brain stem is the *mechanism* of intelligence, but it is not the *source* of it.

We know this because this intelligence exists outside of the human brain stem—it permeates all living organisms. Consider any plant and how it knows to grow without a "brain" telling it what to do or other sentient beings teaching it the way. The sunflower provides an interesting example. Through a process called heliotropism, young sunflowers physically turn their heads to track the sun across the sky from east to west, maximizing their energy intake. At night, they reset to the east, waiting for the sunrise. Who taught the flower to do that? No one. It is the innate intelligence of the organism responding to its environment to ensure survival.

In the animal kingdom, we call this intelligence "instinct"—like the weaver bird's ability to build a nest even when hatched and raised away from older birds[4] and the way the baby kangaroo knows to climb up their mother's stomach after being born to get inside the pouch despite being the size of a jellybean, blind and deaf.

The most convincing proof, however, is your own body. When you cut yourself while cooking, you don't have to sit there and concentrate, telling your blood cells to clot, your white blood cells to rush to the site to fight infection, and your fibroblasts to stitch the skin back together. Your body initiates a complex cascade of thousands of chemical reactions instantly. It knows exactly how to heal itself. The doctor might stitch the wound to hold the edges together, but the doctor doesn't heal the cut. The body does. Similarly, a fever is an intelligent defensive strategy designed to save your life. When the body detects a virus, it realizes that the invader cannot survive in high heat. So, the hypothalamus (the body's thermostat) turns up the temperature to "cook" the virus out.

This is not just biology; it is biology infused with consciousness. It is the Silent Architect at work.

So considering this, it brings us back to the idea that our bodies do not randomly display symptoms that have no cause or meaning—it's far too intelligent for that. Trauma, stress and rigid protective patterns act like a dam in the river, blocking the flow of this intelligence through the spine and creating physical pain. When the answer for the pain is not clear or it's being suppressed or ignored, Spinal Energetics is a tool to access that intelligence through the energetic fields. This intelligence is alive within us all because Spinal Energetics wouldn't work on a dead person—they've got no life force.

Is Spinal Energetics the only way to touch this? No. I believe you can connect with the innate life force through other means too. Meditation as an example. When I was on a 10-day silent Vipassana course, they spoke about this same philosophy, just in a different way. They call it *sankhara*, which are deep-seated emotional impurities, habits, patterns or conditioned reactions that surface as a result of past experiences. They are believed to fuel suffering, but through meditation and with awareness and breath, we can shed these things that are stored and move through them.

I felt the same movement doing these meditations as I did when I do Spinal Energetics. I felt the same inner knowing move through me and felt a deep connection to Source.

So I don't believe that working on the spine is the only way to reach your inner intelligence—it's just one of the ways. Someone who is a Master of Yoga would've experienced a divine connection through postures and working with the breath. However, it takes years of dedication and time to obtain a state of effortless mastery. It's discipline and awareness working together.

But reaching certain levels of mastery in the holistic or spiritual space isn't easily accessible in Western culture. We have been conditioned to instant gratification and for symptoms to be "fixed" rather than understood. Western medicine is often superior for acute and life-saving treatments like heart surgery, broken bones and infections, as it looks through the lens of pathology, anatomy and pharmaceuticals.

Eastern traditions, on the other hand, look at balance and see medicine in a holistic way. They tend to look at patterns and address whole-body wellness over time in a slow and deliberate way using movement, herbs and breathing techniques.

I believe in both.

The Sweet Spot Between East and West

When creating Spinal Energetics, I was aware that the trained Western mind would not want to meditate for two hours like a Vipassana practice. Honestly, who has two hours a fricking day to do that? But nor would an Eastern mind want to neglect the full spectrum of wellness.

I knew that the innate intelligence didn't need mortal time for healing to occur. It operated at a different level and could transform and accelerate change.

So with Spinal Energetics I asked myself: *how can we accelerate people's healing without compromising their process?*

It's similar to the experience people are reporting in plant medicine journeys. How can you take a drink and then a few hours later be a completely transformed person? People are looking for shorter ways to get the result that they would after 20 years of talk therapy. It's an unprecedented change in humanity.

American spiritual teacher of the Tibetan Buddhist lineage, Lama Surya Das, often reminds his students to "meditate as fast as you can"—a playful way to remind people to live mindfully during their fast-paced lives.

The reason fast and remarkable changes can happen is because these methods work directly with the person's awareness and innate intelligence. I personally believe this intelligence lives incubated in our spine because that's where our entire system is held together. There's no point having a brain or a heart without a spine. These organs are complex and incredible, but what's in the middle of them? The spine. It's the highway of life force. The centerpiece that holds all life systems together.

So when we work with the spine, we are trusting that if we enable the body to feel safe, your innate intelligence will take over and do exactly what it has known how to do since the moment you were conceived: **heal, organize and thrive.**

CHAPTER 2

THE LIFE FORCE

UNDERSTANDING THE ENERGY THAT DRIVES US

Now that we understand what our innate intelligence is, it's time to understand the energetic fields that surround us.

Bioelectricity and Electromagnetic Fields

If you look at your hand right now, it appears solid. It has weight, texture, and distinct boundaries. If you clap your hands together, they make a sound. To your senses, and to most of Western medicine, you are a biological machine made of dense matter—bones, muscles, organs, and fluids.

But if we were to look at your hand under a powerful quantum microscope, that solidity would vanish. You would see cells, then molecules, then atoms. And if we looked inside the atom, we would find... almost nothing.

In the simplest of terms, an atom consists of a central nucleus (made of protons and neutrons) and a cloud of electrons. The nucleus sits in the center, while the "outer edge" of the atom is defined by the electrons zipping around at incredible speeds. Because the distance between the nucleus and the electrons is so vast, the atom is 99.9999999% "empty" space.[5] To visualize this, if an atom were the size of a football stadium, the nucleus would be a marble on the 50-yard line and the electrons would be tiny gnats buzzing around the highest nosebleed seats. However, here's the catch: that space isn't actually empty—it is filled with electromagnetic forces.[6] The electrons move so fast that they create a repulsive force field that makes the atom feel solid, much like a spinning propeller looks and feels like a solid disk when in motion.[7] Therefore, we are not solid "things," we are organisms buzzing with energy.

This concept is the foundation of bioelectricity. The science ignited back in 1780 when Italian physician Luigi Galvani touched a spark to a dead frog's leg and watched it kick, proving for the first time that life runs on an electrical current.[8] For centuries, this was viewed as a scientific novelty, but today it is the silent engine of modern healthcare. We no longer just observe these signals; we rely on them to keep us alive. You see this mastery in the pacemaker, a tiny device that uses electrical pulses to override a failing heart, or the cochlear implant, which translates sound waves into electrical signals so deaf people can hear. We have moved beyond seeing the body as a merely chemical structure to understanding it as a complex electrical circuit—one that we are learning not just to read, but to repair.

Epilepsy, for example, is like having too much electricity at once without the ability to disperse it properly, and so it creates seizure activity. Epilepsy is interesting as it presents differently in people. Some develop it later in life while others may have had it since birth. I often see those who have had it since childhood and have found that they are usually highly sensitive and empathetic kids. Since Spinal Energetics is working with the electricity within, we've seen good results with epilepsy, not only with people having fewer seizures but also less intense ones.

On the other side of it, there are those with multiple sclerosis (MS). When using Spinal Energetics over them, it's almost like there's a lag in their bodies' connection, and I think that is because the myelin sheath or the white fatty tissues are affected by MS. When we work with the meninges—which are the three protective membranes that envelop the brain and spinal cord—it's like it takes them longer to "get up and going," but when they do, you can sense a heightened sensitivity there. So in the body, MS can feel slow in movement but with hypervigilant electrical activity. The nervous system is often misfiring its signals due to the damage in the myelin sheath and central nervous system.

We also have an electromagnetic field surrounding us—and the hospital system relies on this fact for several technologies. When you go to the emergency room with chest pain, the first thing they do is an electrocardiogram (ECG). They stick electrodes to your skin to measure the electrical activity of your heart. They are not measuring the heart muscle itself; they are measuring the field of electricity the heart generates.[9]

Similarly, an EEG (electroencephalogram) measures the electrical field of your brain. An MRI (magnetic resonance imaging) uses magnetic fields to interact with the hydrogen atoms in your body to create an image.[10] We accept these medical technologies without question, yet we often reject the underlying premise: that the human body generates, transmits, and is organized by electromagnetic fields.

Research from the HeartMath Institute has shown that the human heart generates the largest electromagnetic field in the body—about 60 times greater in amplitude than the brain's.[11] This field can be measured several feet away from the body using sensitive magnetometers.[12] This means that your "personal space" is physically real. When you stand near someone, your heart's magnetic field is literally overlapping with theirs. This is the scientific basis of "vibes." You aren't imagining that someone feels angry or peaceful; your nervous system is decoding the electromagnetic information broadcast by their heart and brain.

This leads us to the 1940s, when a neuroanatomist at Yale University named Harold Saxton Burr discovered what he called "L-fields" (Life fields).[13] He found that all living things—from salamanders to humans—are surrounded by measurable electromagnetic fields.[14] Crucially, he found that changes in this field preceded changes in the physical body. To prove this, Burr conducted a fascinating series of experiments on mice that were genetically predisposed to breast cancer. Using a sensitive vacuum-tube voltmeter, he tracked the electrical voltage gradients across the animals' bodies over time. He discovered that a significant and chaotic surge in voltage occurred in the specific area where a tumor would later form—roughly two weeks before any lump was palpable or visible. The "L-field" had effectively organized into a pattern of disease before the physical cells had even mutated. This offered the first hard evidence that pathology exists as an energetic disruption before it manifests as a physical reality. He could detect illness in the energy field before it showed up in the cells.[15]

The spine is at the center of that energy system, both structurally through its tensegrity design and electrically through neural conduction. What this means is that disruptions in the biofield can show up as "early warning signals" before disease or dysfunction sets in. When we work in the field around the spine in Spinal Energetics, we may be reorganizing these subtle imbalances before they form into maladaptive neural or physical states or detecting their origin if they've already developed.

The Ancient Practices: Chi, Prana and Chakras

While Western science is just beginning to map this territory, ancient cultures have been navigating it for thousands of years. When combining ancient wisdom with modern science, it becomes apparent that acupuncture is the manipulation of the body's internal current (bioelectricity), whereas modalities like

Reiki or qigong are the manipulation of the external broadcast (the electromagnetic field). What all these things can have in common is that they're working with energy, and even yoga does too. How were the yoga postures even created? How did the Hindus know that certain positions and movements would have certain healing and calming effects? Well, it was developed from energetics.

They may not talk about the quantum field because that wasn't a thing when Buddha was around, but they still understood that the mind, body, consciousness and spiritual components were all connected and that there were energetics behind each posture that would allow the person to shift through the chakras and energy systems via meditation.

In Traditional Chinese Medicine, the body is powered by a vital force called Chi (or Qi). This energy flows through specific channels called meridians. For centuries, Western anatomists dismissed meridians as myth because they could not find them during autopsies. They were looking for distinct tubes, like veins or nerves; however, modern research has revealed that meridians are not tubes; they are pathways of low electrical resistance.

Modern science hypothesizes that the meridians and acupuncture points of Traditional Chinese Medicine align with the fascia network, which is the body's connective tissue, and one study found an 80% correlation between the sites of acupuncture points and the location of intermuscular or intramuscular connective tissue planes.[16] Fascia is a liquid-crystalline matrix that surrounds every muscle and organ, and it is piezoelectric—meaning that when you apply mechanical pressure to it (like inserting a needle), it generates an electrical charge. Therefore, when an acupuncturist inserts a needle into a meridian, they create a micro-electrical surge that travels through the fascial network to the brain, triggering the release of pain-relieving endorphins and regulating the nervous system. They aren't performing magic; they are manipulating the body's bioelectric circuitry.

Healing Without Touch

When it comes to modalities and ancient wisdom that handle the exterior electric field, one of the most common questions is, "How can a person heal someone without touching them?" The answer lies in the physics of induction and resonance. We know from Ampère's Law in physics that any electrical current flowing through a conductor creates a magnetic field around it.[17] Since the human body is running on electrical currents (nerves), it generates a magnetic field (the biofield).

Dr. John Zimmerman measured the magnetic field coming from the hands of trained energy healers using SQUID magnetometers. He found that while a non-healer's hands produced a weak, steady signal, a healer's hands emitted a pulsing magnetic field that swept through frequencies (0.3 to 30 Hz) known to stimulate tissue repair.[18]

This is the principle of entrainment. Entrainment is the process of independent rhythms interacting and influencing each other, resulting in synchronization.[19]

This phenomenon was first noticed in 1666 by Dutch physicist Christian Huygens, the inventor of the pendulum clock. He discovered the principle of entrainment while confined to his room due to illness. Huygens observed that two pendulum clocks hanging on the same beam had synchronized their swings, moving in opposite directions.

Huygens realized that things that should technically operate independently could "sympathize" with each other and sync into a common and stable rhythm. Even when the clocks were started at different times, they would eventually synchronize, with the "faster" clock slowing down and the "slower" clock speeding up until they met at a joint speed.

The explanation for this phenomenon is that very small amounts of energy are transferred between the two objects when their vibrations or frequencies are not the same. The energy transfer forces the two objects to start vibrating and resonating at the same pace. In short, the weaker system becomes entrained by the stronger system.

You can see this in nature when fireflies flash in unison or schools of fish swim as "one."

Our bodies are also full of natural rhythms, like our breathing, heart rate, digestion and sleep cycles. We are electromagnetic creatures with biological rhythms. We influence and affect each other.[20]

Just as a large, vibrating tuning fork will cause a smaller, silent tuning fork to start vibrating if brought near it, a practitioner with a coherent, regulated biofield can "entrain" the chaotic, stressed field of a client. Entrainment enables an organized electromagnetic field to reorganize a disorganized one.

Deborah's Case Study

I had a client called Deborah come into our clinic. She was exhausted, fragile and on the verge of burnout. She was a mother, a wife, a business owner and president of a not-for-profit initiative. To say she was spreading herself thin is an understatement. Deborah collapsed on the table like it was the only place she'd ever rested. I could immediately sense her body was drained and her anxiety was high. Using the principle of entrainment, I rhythmically worked within the field to help her body recognize its natural "home" of sync and coherence. It wasn't that she was doing anything "wrong," it was just that her body and mind became dysregulated and oscillated out of sync.

Energy Fields Within

In Ayurvedic and Yogic traditions, the energy anatomy is detailed and precise. Within the biofield, the Yogis mapped seven primary energy centers called chakras. While these are often depicted in New Age art as colorful spinning flowers, they are, in reality, maps of the human neuro-endocrine system. Every chakra corresponds to a major nerve plexus (a massive bundle of nerves) and a major endocrine gland. They are the transducers of the body—the biological gearboxes that turn "energy" (a thought or emotion) into "matter" (hormones and chemistry).

When we look at the function of these glands, we realize that the ancient "spiritual" descriptions were actually accurate physiological observations:

- **The Root Chakra (Muladhara)—The Adrenal Glands**
    - ~ **The yogic view:** This center governs our instinct for survival, safety and grounding.
    - ~ **The physiology:** This aligns with the adrenal glands, which sit atop the kidneys. The adrenals are responsible for the "fight or flight" response, releasing cortisol and adrenaline when we feel threatened.
    - ~ **The correlation:** When your root chakra is described as "blocked" or "overactive" in yoga, it essentially means you are stuck in a chronic sympathetic nervous system response. You aren't just "spiritually ungrounded"; you are chemically flooded with stress hormones, unable to switch off your survival drive.

- **The Sacral Chakra (Svadhisthana)—The Gonads (Ovaries/Testes)**
    - ~ **The yogic view:** This center governs creativity, sexuality, pleasure and our ability to "flow" with life.
    - ~ **The physiology:** This corresponds to the reproductive

glands (ovaries and testes), which produce estrogen, progesterone and testosterone. These hormones control not just reproduction, but also emotional swings and physical vitality.

- ~ **The correlation:** Biologically, creation and procreation are the same mechanism. The biological drive to create life (reproduction) is the same energy required to create art or new ideas. When this center is balanced, our hormonal cycles regulate our mood and our capacity for connection.

- **The Solar Plexus (Manipura)—The Pancreas**
  - ~ **The yogic view:** This is the center of personal power, will, self-esteem, and "gut instincts." It is the fire in the belly.
  - ~ **The physiology:** This aligns with the pancreas and the celiac plexus. The pancreas releases insulin and enzymes to digest food and convert it into fuel (glucose) for the body.
  - ~ **The correlation:** Just as the pancreas digests physical matter to create energy for the body, the solar plexus "digests" life experiences to create energy for the personality. It is the engine room. If you cannot metabolize your food, you have no physical energy; if you cannot metabolize your life experiences (trauma/stress), you have no personal power.

- **The Heart Chakra (Anahata)—The Thymus Gland**
  - ~ **The yogic view:** This is the center of love and compassion and the bridge between the physical and spiritual self.
  - ~ **The physiology:** This corresponds to the thymus gland, located in the center of the chest. The thymus is the training academy for T-Cells, which are the soldiers of the immune system.
  - ~ **The correlation:** The immune system's job is to distinguish "Self" from "Non-Self." It protects you. In biology, immunity is the ultimate act of self-love and preservation. It is no coincidence that grief and heartbreak—emotional states of the heart chakra—are scientifically proven to suppress the immune system.

- **The Throat Chakra (Vishuddha)—The Thyroid Gland**
  - ~ **The yogic view:** This center governs communication, expression and speaking one's truth.
  - ~ **The physiology:** This aligns with the thyroid gland in the throat. The thyroid produces thyroxine, which regulates metabolism—the rate at which your body burns energy to function.
  - ~ **The correlation:** Expression is essentially the act of turning internal energy into external reality (sound/ speech). When we hold back our truth or repress our expression, we are literally stifling our metabolic output. A "blocked" throat often manifests physically as thyroid

dysfunction—a metabolism that is either running too hot (anxiety/speaking too much) or too cold (depression/silence).

- **The Third Eye (Ajna)—The Pituitary Gland**
  - ~ **The yogic view:** This is the center of intuition, insight and "inner knowing." It is the command center.
  - ~ **The physiology:** This corresponds to the pituitary gland, often called the "Master Gland." It sits deep in the brain and sends chemical instructions to almost every other gland in the body, telling them when to release hormones.
  - ~ **The correlation:** Just as the pituitary allows the brain to control the body's chemistry, the Third Eye allows the mind to perceive the bigger picture. It is the control tower. When the ancient texts said this center "sees all," they were describing the biological reality of the gland that monitors and regulates the entire system.

- **The Crown Chakra (Sahasrara)—The Pineal Gland**
  - ~ **The yogic view:** This center governs spirituality, enlightenment and our connection to the divine/universal consciousness.
  - ~ **The physiology:** This aligns with the pineal gland, a tiny pinecone-shaped structure deep in the brain. It produces melatonin and regulates our circadian rhythms (sleep/wake cycles) based on the detection of light.

- **The correlation:** The pineal gland literally regulates our relationship with light. In almost every spiritual tradition, the divine is described as "The Light." Biologically, this gland allows us to sync our internal biological clock with the external cycles of the universe (the sun and moon). It is our physical interface with the cosmos.

Each of these seven centers is not just a gland; it is a massive intersection of nerve endings (a plexus). Because nerves operate on electrical impulses, these areas are regions of incredibly high bioelectrical voltage compared to the rest of the body. Going back to Ampère's Law—where there is an electric current, there is a magnetic field—we can see that these seven high-voltage intersections naturally generate seven distinct electromagnetic fields that project outward from the spine. When the ancient mystics saw "spinning wheels" of energy, they were visualizing the electromagnetic turbulence generated by these powerful nerve plexuses. Therefore, when a practitioner senses a "block" in the field above your stomach, they aren't imagining it; they are literally feeling the magnetic distortion caused by electrical stress in your solar plexus and pancreas. The "aura" is simply the sum total of these seven biological broadcasts.

The Language Gap

When I was practicing Reiki, what I didn't love was the use of language when something was considered "blocked." I think it makes people feel bad about themselves. No one has consciously blocked one of their chakras—it's unconscious. And additionally, it's not tangible. It's like an idea in the sky. And then, the facilitator might say, "I'm going to unblock it for you." That's placing the power on the practitioner.

Don't get me wrong, Reiki is amazing and working with the chakras is important, that's why we utilize them as well, but Spinal Energetics has a very different approach and philosophy to it. Saying something is blocked or stuck reinforces the idea that the body's done something wrong. Whereas in my opinion, if it has been blocked or stuck, we use words like it's disconnected or in a protective mode. And that gives meaning to the reason why the body has responded that way. The body is wise and has done something for a good cause.

Most importantly, my goal isn't to unblock something if the body has blocked it. My goal is to create safety so that protective strategy or disconnection can be seen and the body can resolve it on its own.

"Natural forces within us are the true healers of disease."

Hippocrates

For thousands of years, the language gap kept these worlds apart. The mystic spoke of "blocks in the Nadis," while the doctor spoke of "impingement in the nerves." The healer spoke of a "weak aura," while the physicist spoke of "low amplitude electromagnetic oscillation." Today, we now understand that the bioelectricity discovered by Galvani is the Chi described by the Taoists and the electromagnetic field is the aura seen by the yogis.

Understanding the energetic field moves us from a mechanic's view of the body to a gardener's view. A mechanic fixes parts; a gardener tends to the soil, the light and the water, knowing that the plant has the intelligence to grow itself.

Your biofield is the soil. Your spine is the stem. Your innate intelligence is the force of life driving the growth. When we honor all three—the science, the spirit and the structure—we unlock a potential for healing that is limitless.

CHAPTER 3

The Connection Between Our Emotional and Physical Fields

Now that we have two out of the three fundamental truths that make up Spinal Energetics, it's time to tackle the third: our emotional and physical fields are interconnected, so what affects us emotionally manifests physically and vice versa. The mind–body connection isn't woo-woo; it's basic science. Think of your everyday mind–body connection like "butterflies in the tummy," your cheeks blushing from embarrassment, and sleep disturbances due to stress or worry. As the great Joseph Pilates once said, "The mind and body are not separate. What affects one, affects the other."

The understanding of the mind–body connection has gone mainstream, with thousands of peer-reviewed scientific articles from different industries revealing the intrinsic link between them, including neuroscience,[21] psychology, sport science, Yoga, meditation, arts,[22] and allied health services.[23]

The fact that mental and physical health are intimately linked cannot be overlooked or pushed aside. Current research has found that mental and physical illnesses frequently occur in tandem,[24] and furthermore, psychosocial issues such as adverse experiences, stress and emotional upheaval have profound influences on a person's health and well-being.[25]

So what happens when you go to the doctor and they can't find a physical reason for your pain or symptoms? They often shrug their shoulders, give you painkillers and tell you to come back if the pain doesn't go away on its own. That's because Western medical training often neglects the mind–body understanding and puts conditions into separate boxes: physical and mental. This is not the doctors' fault as they are under enough pressure, it just means that most first-contact doctors do not have all the tools to see that physical symptoms could potentially be driven by the emotional or mental aspects of the patient.

Take chronic pain for example. Pain is a modern epidemic with an estimated 20% of adults suffering from pain globally, with 10% being newly diagnosed with chronic pain each year.[26] That's a lot of people suffering unnecessarily.

The Australian 2024 National Pain Report revealed that 72.9% of adult pain sufferers have felt ignored or dismissed when raising their pain with health professionals.[27] And a whopping 9 in 10 young people living with pain report being ignored or dismissed by health professionals.[28]

If we look at pain *only* through a physical lens, then those numbers reveal that most people suffering from pain are not being adequately treated, listened to or taken seriously. They are left to suffer in silence on their own.

With a more holistic view, these people can have more options of treatment.

To understand how a holistic approach can help treat physical pain, let's look at the different types of physical ailments:

- **Purely physical:** These are acute injuries or bodily traumas resulting from direct external force or immediate physiological damage, like breaking an arm, cutting yourself while cooking, or getting into a trauma accident.
- **Emotional pain with physical manifestations:** These are somatic responses where intense psychological distress or prolonged internal pressure translates into tangible biological symptoms and illnesses. Think getting a tight chest when severely anxious, breaking out in shingles when stressed, or developing an autoimmune disease from trauma or extended periods of stress/high cortisol release.
- **Conditions that are physical in nature but have emotional variables:** These are physiological diseases that originate independently of your mental state but are significantly modulated by your psychological well-being, like diabetes, some types of cancer and chronic illnesses.

> While they have developed on a purely physical plane, your mental state can influence your management of the symptoms. When you are more stressed, anxious or depressed, your symptoms can spiral out of control, but when you are looking after your mental health, you feel in control and your symptoms return to manageable levels.

Even when we have a purely physical injury, like breaking an arm, it has ramifications for our mental health because of the pain, possible trauma around the event and hospital system, and the limitations in daily life. And so when we suffer from a mental injury, like grief, it makes sense that the physical aspect of our bodies also reacts. And yet this connection between our mental and physical states is something that Westerners in particular grapple with.

To understand why your lower back aches when you are financially stressed or why your neck seizes up when you cannot speak your truth, we must bridge the gap between the world of matter and the world of energy. We must understand the connection between our mental fields and our physical vessels. We must evolve beyond the rudimentary aspects of "parts" and look at the whole rather than just the sum of parts. As Plato reminded us centuries ago, "The cure of the part should not be attempted without treatment of the whole."

Belief and Biology

For years, we believed we were victims of our genetics—that our DNA was a fixed destiny. But cellular biologist Dr. Bruce Lipton challenged this dogma with a groundbreaking insight. His early research—suggesting that the environment of the cell determines its fate, not just the genetics—paved the path for what is now a cornerstone of modern biology: epigenetics. This is the study of how environment and behavior turn genes on and off without changing the DNA sequence itself.[29]

Lipton discovered that the cell's membrane acts like a sensory organ. It reads environmental signals and communicates with the DNA to alter gene expression.[30] This means that genes do not control our biology in isolation; instead, they are influenced by signals from outside the cell.

This provides the biological bridge between mind and matter: our thoughts, emotions, and beliefs generate specific neurochemical signals (like cortisol or dopamine) that travel to the cell membrane and actively influence how our genes express themselves. In other words, our bodies can be retrained by changing our internal environment.

Dr. Lipton's biology of belief suggests that regardless of the genetic hand you were dealt, you possess the capacity to shift how those genes express themselves in the present. There is, of course, a scientific distinction to be made here: you cannot "think" your way into changing your eye color or erasing a fixed chromosomal defect (like Down syndrome). You cannot change the hard-coded DNA sequence. However, you *can* change the DNA expression.

Since gene activity is heavily influenced by the cellular environment (stress, diet, toxins), and that environment is regulated by your neurochemistry (cortisol versus dopamine), shifting your internal state directly influences your physical health.[31]

Consider how this works in practice. If your mind perceives a threat—whether it is a tiger chasing you or a toxic work environment—the biological response is identical.[32] Your brain floods the system with stress hormones like cortisol and adrenaline. These chemicals wash over your cells, forcing them into a state of "protection." Crucially, biology dictates that a cell cannot be in growth and protection at the same time. To conserve energy for the perceived battle, your cells stop repairing tissue, maintaining the body, or reproducing. They also downregulate the immune system.[33] If this stress becomes chronic, your nervous system is essentially locking your cells in a permanent defensive stance, and inevitably, the mental field (the belief that you are unsafe) creates a direct physical consequence (inflammation, suppressed immunity, and cellular decay) due to the compromised immune system.[34]

So what does this mean for Spinal Energetics? It means that we can use this practice to read what is happening on this cellular level so that you can make changes to your life that will improve your physical symptoms.

Sage's Case Study

I once had a client, Sage, who was suffering from chronic bronchitis. She was prescribed a variety of medications by various doctors, but they couldn't figure out why it kept recurring. She came to me as a last resort (as many clients do). After chatting for quite some time, I worked with her energetically.

Her body was fatigued but in the field I received an intuitive hit that signified her body's stress was somehow related to her career direction. I said to her, "There seems to be a misalignment between you and your career." That's not a huge misalignment for everyone, but for certain people, their career is a large expression of who they are in the world. Sage was one of those people.

She said, "Yeah, I hate my job. I'm sick of being there, but I need the money." I asked her what she found the hardest part about working there. "Well, my boss never listens to me. He never listens to anything I say. It's like I'm speaking and he hears nothing."

She didn't realize that she was voicing the answer to her constant bronchitis. She went on to tell me that no one listened to her growing up and this issue was now happening in her adult life. She said that she was "sick and tired of it."

I said, "I think there's possibly a connection with your chronic bronchitis and your environment. The reason I sense this is because you keep going back into the same environment over and over again, so the body is getting louder, like announcing to you, 'Hey Sage, you need to pay attention to this.'"

She hadn't even considered they could be linked. She took four months of long-service leave and didn't get bronchitis once.

It's important to note here that it wasn't the spinal work that healed the bronchitis, but it was what showed the misalignment between her career and her symptoms. She was in an environment that suppressed her voice, and so her cells reflected that suppression with a physical ailment that did the same thing.

Psychological stress is a recognized risk factor for upper respiratory infections (like acute bronchitis) and can trigger flare-ups of chronic respiratory conditions.[35] Several studies have also shown that childhood adversity is associated with an increased risk of stress-related physical health outcomes, such as asthma and chronic bronchitis later in life.[36]

She ended up moving jobs and hasn't had bronchitis since. That doesn't mean she won't ever get it again. Maybe there will be another time in her life when her voice gets suppressed and the same thing will show up, especially since there's a susceptibility there now. But what Spinal Energetics does is bridge the patterns between the emotional issue and the physical response. It helps uncover and reveal relationships between the physical manifestations and the mental and emotional states.

The Pharmacy Within

Dr. Lipton's theoretical framework has been expanded by Dr. Joe Dispenza, a researcher and author who has dedicated his career to demystifying the mind–body connection. While Lipton provided the biology, Dispenza provided the method, backed by extensive data collected from thousands of brain scans and blood tests.

His core thesis is simple but radical: **You are your own pharmacy.**

Dispenza explains that the brain and body communicate through a continuous feedback loop. He states, "Thoughts are the language of the brain, and feelings are the language of the body."[37] The moment you have a thought—for example, remembering a painful argument—your brain releases a specific chemical signature (neuropeptides) that signals the body to feel the corresponding emotion. Within seconds, you feel the heat of anger or the knot of anxiety.

The body then sends a signal back to the brain: "I am feeling angry." The brain, monitoring the body, says, "Oh, we are angry? I should think more angry thoughts to match that state."

This creates a state of being. The problem arises when this loop becomes chronic. If you think fearful thoughts and feel fearful emotions every day for years, your body becomes chemically addicted to that cocktail of stress hormones. You may intellectually *want* to be happy, but your body is craving the rush of cortisol and adrenaline because that is its baseline. As Dispenza puts it, the body has literally "become the mind"—it is running the show on autopilot.

In one of his advanced workshops, Dispenza sought to prove that we can upgrade our immune system by changing our internal state. He took blood samples from 120 subjects before the workshop to measure their levels of Immunoglobulin A (IgA)—the body's primary defense against bacteria and viruses. He then asked the participants to practice a specific meditation where they moved into a state of "heart coherence"—sustaining elevated emotions like gratitude and love for 10 minutes, three times a day. After four days, he re-tested their blood. The results were staggering: average IgA levels had shot up by 50 percent.[38] There was no change in diet or medication; the only variable was their emotional state. By simply changing their internal "signal" from survival (stress) to creation (gratitude), they significantly upregulated their genetic expression for immunity.

In Spinal Energetics, we see this mind–body connection manifested in the spine. The spine is the main highway of the central nervous system. It carries the signals between the brain and the body. When we are stuck in negative loops—when we are living by the hormones of stress—the spine becomes rigid. The energy stops flowing. The "current" gets blocked.

We often see clients who have done years of talk therapy. They understand their trauma intellectually. They can tell you exactly why they are the way they are, but they are still in pain. Why? Because while they changed their minds, they didn't change their energy. As Dr. Dispenza paraphrases from Einstein, "We cannot think our way out of a problem with the same mind that created it."[39] We have to enter the body and the energetic field to break the cycle.

Stephanie's Case Study

One client I worked with, let's call her Stephanie, had spent over a decade in various forms of traditional talk therapy. She was articulate, psychologically insightful, and deeply self aware. She could trace her patterns back to early childhood, name the very formative moments, and explain her emotional responses with such clarity. From the outside, it looked like "the work" had been done.

Yet her body told a completely different story.

She lived with a persistent tension through her neck and chest, chronic fatigue, shallow breathing, and a background sense of anxiety that never quite went away. Despite understanding her "trauma," her nervous system still responded as though the threat was ongoing. Her body remained in a subtle but constant state of mobilization.

When she began Spinal Energetics, the shifts were not conceptual, they were physiological. In the early sessions, her body exhibited involuntary responses: changes in breath, spontaneous muscular release through the spine, and periods of deep parasympathetic settling. These responses were not something she was "trying" to do nor was she "performing." They were reflexive, emerging as the nervous system moved out of long-held protective patterns.

What surprised her most was not having to re-live her past experiences consciously and yet experience both an emotional release and a reorganization. Over time, she noticed that she no longer lived in the same background tension. Situations that previously activated her sympathetic nervous system now registered differently in her body. The narrative of her trauma had not changed, but her relationship to it had. Her physiology no longer reacted as if the past was happening in the present moment.

This is where many people reach the limit of purely cognitive approaches. Insight can create understanding, but the nervous system learns through experience. When the body is given a new reference point of safety and coherence, the old patterns begin to lose their charge and not because they are "overcome," but because the system no longer needs to organize itself around them.

The Body Knows

Perhaps the most profound validation of the somatic (body-based) approach comes from the work of Dr. Bessel van der Kolk, one of the world's leading experts on traumatic stress. In his seminal work, *The Body Keeps the Score*, he moved the conversation beyond psychology and into neurology, detailing how trauma is not just a historical event but a physiological imprint left on the brain and body.[40]

Van der Kolk did not just theorize this; he captured it in real time. In the early 1990s at Harvard, Van der Kolk and his team conducted a landmark study using PET scans on patients with PTSD.[41] They wanted to see what happens to the brain when a person recalls a traumatic event. They placed participants in the scanner and played back audio scripts of their specific traumas.

What the scans revealed was shocking. As the patients entered a state of recall, their emotional brains (the limbic system) lit up with intense activity, signaling high arousal. But simultaneously, a specific region in the left frontal lobe called Broca's Area went completely dark.

Broca's Area is the speech center of the brain. It is responsible for translating thoughts into words. The scans showed that during a trauma response, the brain literally loses the physical capacity to speak and articulate the experience. The participants were not being stubborn; their brains had experienced a partial shutdown similar to that of a stroke victim.

This experiment provided the scientific explanation for "speechless terror." It proved that trauma is stored in the non-verbal, emotional right brain, while the capacity to explain it lives in the logical left brain. When the trauma is activated, the bridge between the two collapses.

This is why traditional talk therapy can hit a wall. You cannot "talk" your way out of a state when the speech center is offline. You cannot use logic to reorganize an experience that is being held in the primitive, survival parts of the brain. And because the mind cannot process the event verbally, the energy of the experience is relegated to the body. Van der Kolk argues that the body "keeps the score" in the form of a recalibrated nervous system.[42] The brain of a traumatized person is constantly mistaking the present for the past, signaling the body to remain in a state of high alert.

The memory is preserved not as a story, but as a physical sensation: a clenched jaw, a frozen shoulder, a churn in the gut, or a spine that curves under the weight of invisible burdens. Van der Kolk concludes that we need more than top-down approaches to heal (using thoughts to change feelings). We need bottom-up approaches—methods that start with the body to reset the brainstem and the autonomic nervous system.

In Spinal Energetics, we apply this bottom-up principle. By

engaging the nervous system directly through the spine and the energetic field, we bypass the "offline" speech centers and speak directly to the body, allowing it to release the tension it has been holding since the original event.

In my practice, I have seen this time and time again. I will be working on a client's spine, perhaps gently influencing a blockage in the thoracic region—the area often associated with the heart center and emotional expression—and suddenly, the client will begin to weep. They aren't crying because of physical pain. They are crying because the energy of a decade-old grief, held tightly in the fascia and musculature of their back, is finally being given permission to move.

The physical release allows for the emotional release. The mental field and the physical field are unlocking each other.

When the Body Says No

But what happens if we don't listen? What happens if we ignore the tension, the anxiety, and the subtle whispers of our intuition?

Dr. Gabor Maté, a renowned physician and expert in palliative care, suggests that when we are unable to say "no" to the demands of others—when we suppress our authenticity to maintain attachment—our bodies say "no" for us. This "no" manifests as disease.[43]

Maté's conclusions are drawn from decades of clinical observation in family practice and palliative care. He noticed a startling pattern among his most critically ill patients, particularly those with autoimmune diseases, cancer and ALS. They were not angry or difficult people; in fact, they were often the opposite. They were the caregivers, the peacemakers and the stoics. They were the people who never complained and always put others' needs before their own.

Maté argues that this "niceness" is often a survival strategy developed in childhood—a suppression of healthy aggression to avoid rejection. While this saves the relationship, it destroys the biology. To validate this, Maté points to the pioneering work of researcher Lydia Temoshok at the University of California, San Francisco. Temoshok identified a specific behavior pattern she called the Type C personality: individuals who are cooperative, unassertive, patient and who suppress negative emotions (particularly anger).

In her studies of melanoma (skin cancer) patients, Temoshok found a direct biological correlation. She measured the activity of the patients' Natural Killer (NK) cells—the immune system's specialized soldiers responsible for attacking tumors and viruses. The results were undeniable: the patients who repressed their emotions (Type C) had significantly weaker NK cell activity.[44] Because they were psychologically "standing down" and suppressing their defense mechanisms to please others, their immune systems mimicked that state, literally "standing down" at a cellular level and allowing the cancer to spread.[45]

This links to the broader field of psychoneuroimmunology (PNI)—the study of how the mind, nervous system, and immune system interact. PNI has established that the repression of emotion triggers a chronic stress response.[46] By burying anger or grief, the body is forced to maintain a high-level physiological load to keep that energy contained. This floods the system with cortisol, which, over time, desensitizes the immune receptors and confuses the body's ability to distinguish between "self" and "invader."

As Maté famously states, "The question is not what is wrong with the body, but what is the body trying to say?"[47]

In Spinal Energetics, we view the spine as the place where these "unsaid no's" are stored. The rigid posture of a client often reflects years of "holding it together." By facilitating the release of this stored tension, we are not just relaxing muscles; we are helping the nervous system finally express the boundary it was never allowed to set, thereby freeing the immune system to return to its job of protecting the body.

“The body knows things about which the mind is ignorant.”

JACQUES LECOQ

CHAPTER 4

THE SPINE AS THE AXIS

This brings us back to the spine.

Why the spine? Why is this the focal point of our work?

In Spinal Energetics, we view the spine as the primary antenna of the body. Biologically, the spine houses the spinal cord and is the superhighway of information that connects your brain to every single organ, tissue, and cell in your body. It is the master controller. If there is interference in the spine, there is interference in the signal to the stomach, the heart, the lungs and the legs.

But energetically, the spine is the central channel (the Sushumna in yoga) through which your innate intelligence flows. When we experience trauma—physical, emotional or chemical—it disrupts this flow.

If the trauma is too much to process, the system "pauses" it and stores the energy as tension, not just in the muscles, but in the field itself. It creates a distortion in the blueprint. This is why physical manipulation alone sometimes fails. You can crack the bone back into place (fixing the particle), but if the energetic tension (the wave) remains in the field, it will simply pull the bone back out of alignment. The pattern hasn't changed.

Working With the Five Energetic Layers

In a Spinal Energetics session, we interact with these different layers of the field to access the innate intelligence.

- **Physical:** A physical, structural injury or tension.
- **Mental:** A story that has been created and perpetuated, keeping the psychology stuck and in a loop (a limiting belief, for example). Interacting with the biofield—the electromagnetic bubble where the "memory" of the stress is held.
- **Emotional:** Unprocessed and suppressed emotions that become stuck.
- **Spiritual:** An empathetic load of sorts, perhaps carrying a burden, trauma or emotion for someone else, like a partner or parent.
- **Personal Soul:** The authentic self—a disconnect between what the soul needs and what the reality is, or a lesson that is connected to growth.

When we view the spine through the lens of Spinal Energetics, we are reading a story. We are reading where you have held on, where you have let go, where you are frozen in the past, and where you are anxious about the future. By bringing awareness and resonance to these subtle layers, we are essentially sending a new signal to the brain. We are saying, "Pay attention here. There is static in the signal."

Because the field dictates the matter, when we clear the resistance in the energy field, the physical body follows. The muscles relax, the breath deepens, and the spine self-corrects. We are not forcing the spine straight; we are clearing the interference so the innate intelligence can straighten it for us.

We can return to a state of flow.

The spine is not only structural, but also the gateway of energy, optimal health and energy. It is a living thing that combines your physical, mental, emotional and spiritual self.

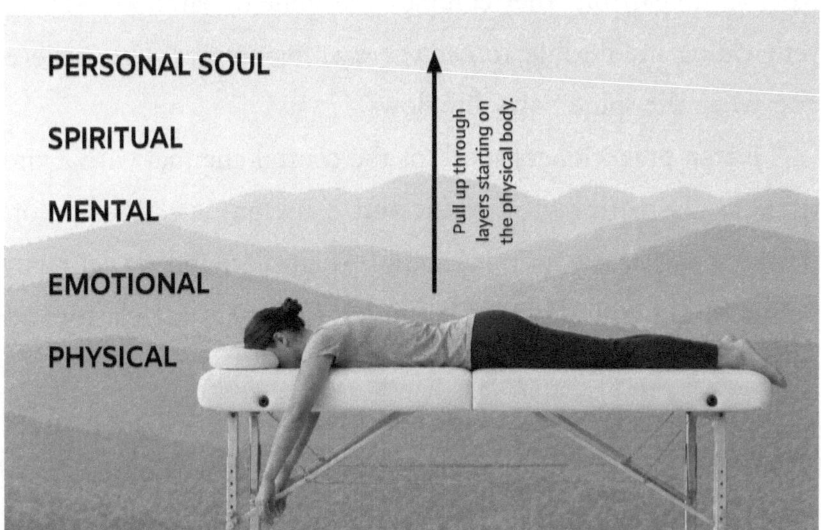

Ancient Ideas with Modern Science

Let's be honest, I am not the first to point to the spine as the axis. Ancient traditions and cultures have long seen the spine as more than vertebrae and nerves. Way before anatomy textbooks existed, cultures across the globe mapped the spine as the body's central axis—not only structurally, but spiritually, emotionally, and cosmologically.

In the yogic traditions of India, the spine is the sacred channel of spiritual awakening. At its base rests Kundalini, the coiled potential of life itself. The Yogic practice considers that when the spine is aligned and the breath steady, energy ascends, and awareness expands. The human being becomes a bridge between awareness and illumination.

In Taoist practice, the spine is a river of Qi. The Governing Vessel (Du Mai) carries vitality to the brain and back down again in the great circulation known in their tradition as the Microcosmic Orbit. They compare the spine to bamboo—strong yet yielding and flexible; rooted yet reaching upward. They believe that when the spine flows, life flows.

Tibetan practitioners speak of the central channel within the spine as the pathway of winds and consciousness. Meditation postures emphasize a "vajra spine"—dignified and upright but not tense. The spine becomes a conduit for inner heat, clarity, and awakening. Stability of posture feeds the stability of mind.

Indigenous cultures across the world echo this same pattern. The human spine reflects the World Tree—the axis mundi connecting earth below and sky above. Shamans journey along this invisible ladder. In Andean traditions, energy centers along the spine relate to levels of perception and relationship—to self, community, nature, and cosmos. It's a sacred column that connects self to life, and to lose alignment is to lose connection. To restore the spine is to restore connection.

In Western osteopathy and chiropractic traditions, the language shifts but the understanding remains. The spine is the highway of the nervous system. Structure governs function. So, when the spine moves uninhibited and freely, communication between brain and body is restored. Modern somatics like Spinal Energetics adds another layer: the spine is also shaped by experiences. Trauma, resilience, grief, and joy all leave impressions along its length.

Even everyday language in society involves the spine. People say cowards are "spineless," or that "to have a spine" is to stand in truth and "have a backbone."

These common threads place the spine as the center of life and as the conduit and channel of life and matter. Perhaps this is why so many practices—yoga, qigong, dance, prayer, meditation, breathwork—return again and again to the same instruction: lengthen upward, root downward, soften in the middle. Feel the axis. Become aware of the central line.

To work with the spine, in any culture, is to work with alignment—of body, energy, and meaning. It is to remember that we are built around a center. And that when that center is clear, life moves more freely through us.

In the coming chapters, we will explore exactly how this works, how the different layers of the energetic field interact, and how you can begin to listen to the language of your own body. But for now, let this be your foundation: You are not a machine. You are a vast, interconnected field of intelligence. And your body is always, always on your side, waiting for you to listen.

In Spinal Energetics, we are reading a story.

We are reading where you have held on, where you have let go, where you are frozen in the past, and where you are anxious about the future.

PART TWO

THE LANGUAGE OF THE SPINE

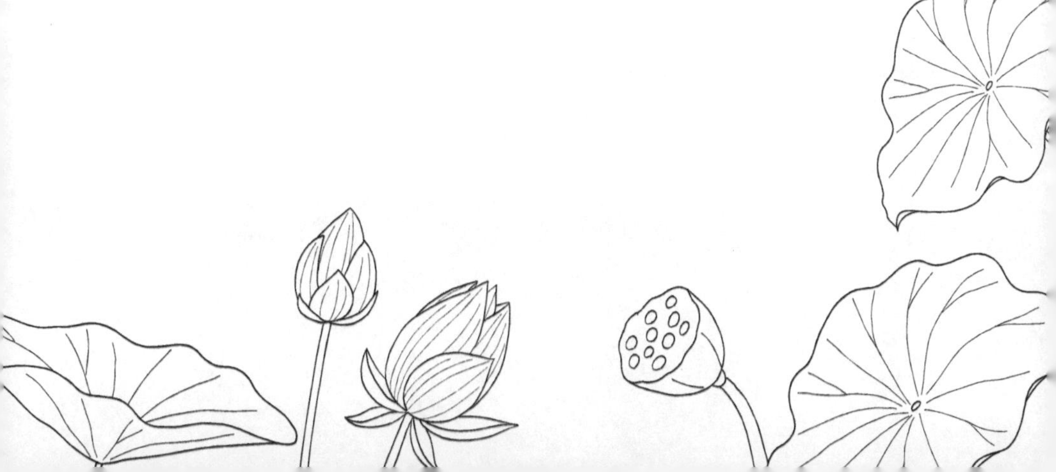

CHAPTER 5

THE SPINE HOLDS YOUR STORY

Spinal Energetics is not a technique to fix you, but an experience to reveal you.

Your spine holds your story. It holds the memories you have forgotten, the tension of the words you never spoke, and the potential you have yet to express.

To understand just how vital and protective the spine is, we only need to look at how certain viruses interact with it. Consider the herpes virus, which causes cold sores. Medical science struggles to find a permanent cure for it. Why? Because the virus is intelligent enough to retreat into the spine. It knows that the spine is the ultimate sanctuary—untouchable and protected. If the immune system were to launch a full-scale attack on the virus while it was hiding in the spinal cord, it could cause catastrophic damage to the host. So, the body allows it to stay. Just as a virus can lie dormant there for years only to flare up when the system is stressed, your spine holds dormant emotions, old traumas and even protective strategies.

When we look at the spine solely as a structural object, we miss the narratives living inside it. We miss the fact that the posture you hold is often a shape you adopted to survive a past version of your life.

Take scoliosis, for example. In the medical world, we often attribute the development of scoliosis in young teenage girls to hormonal changes during puberty. And while the biology is valid, there is often a spiritual or energetic layer that coincides with it. It is usually diagnosed at the exact time a young girl is becoming a woman—a time when she is suddenly compressed by the weight of societal expectations, the gaze of the world, and the pressure to fit into a box that may not fit her soul. I have often wondered if the spine curves and twists not just because of hormones, but because the spirit is physically compressing itself against the alignment of a world it doesn't feel safe in.

Even the way we enter the world impacts this spinal connection. When we interfere with the innate intelligence of the spine during birth—for example, with the use of an epidural—we alter the communication channel. An epidural is designed to block pain, which is often necessary and merciful, but it also blocks the innate connection between mother and child during the most critical moment of their meeting. You can no longer feel the baby moving and shifting in the same way; you are pushing because you are told to, not because you feel the urge. We numb the pain, but in doing so, we numb the wisdom. This is not to say there isn't a wonderful place for modern medicine—it's simply to show the incredible work of the spine. The fact it holds all our experiences and sends vital messages to us in every phase of our lives, from birth to death.

This is often how we treat our spines throughout our lives: we seek to numb the sensation, thinking it's just physical pain, rather than listening to the message. But your spine does not signal pain for no reason and it shouldn't be a storage unit overflowing with past traumas and unhelpful behaviors. At first, it will quietly ask you to listen with a twinge or an ache. If you do not listen to this whisper, it will scream louder and louder until you finally do.

How the Spine Speaks Its Story

You likely already know the language of your spine, even if you haven't had the words to translate it yet. The body is incredibly literal in its expression. It expresses what the mind represses.

When we look at a client, we are not just looking for alignment in the chiropractic sense; we are looking for the story. The posture itself—the curvatures, the tension points, the way a person holds themselves—is a reflection of how they are functioning in life.

We tend to think of posture as a purely mechanical result of our modern lives. We tell ourselves that we hunch because we sit at desks all day or that our necks are sore because we spend too much time looking down at our phones. And while our environment certainly plays a role, to view posture as solely physical is to miss the majority of the story.

Your posture—the way you hold yourself, the curvature of your spine, the tone of your muscles—is a direct reflection of how you are functioning in life. It is the language of your history, your trauma, your beliefs, and your emotional state, frozen in time.

We know this intuitively. If someone walks into a dinner party hunched over, eyes downcast, and shoulders rolled forward, you immediately sense a story of defeat, hiding, or sadness. Conversely, if someone enters with their chest open, chin up, and stride fluid, you perceive confidence and vitality. Harvard researchers have even quantified this, famously studying "power postures" and discovering that simply holding a stance of confidence can alter the testosterone and cortisol levels in the blood.[48] But I think it's also vice versa. Not only can we change our physiology by changing our posture purposely, but our physiology impacts the way we're functioning and that presents in our posture.

Spinal Energetics looks at the spine as a map of archetypes. When a client walks into my clinic, I am already reading the autobiography of their energy field before they have even said hello. I am looking at where they are holding on, where they are letting go, where they are protecting themselves, and where they have disconnected. Here are the insights into the pattern of stories of the spine.

Spinal Energetics is reading the autobiography of their energy field.

The Lower Back (Lumbar) – The Foundation

Structure: The lumbar spine is the lower back, and it consists of five durable vertebrae (L1–L5) situated between the thoracic spine and the sacrum. The lumbar is designed to support upper body weight, allow movement, and protect the lower spinal cord. It is meant to have a lordotic curve (a gentle inward sway).

Energetic center: The lower back is the domain of the solar plexus and the sacral chakras. We use the energetic centers as momentum to work with the spinal tension pattern. We typically use the solar plexus for the lower back.

Relational language: This area is deeply connected to our sense of safety, survival, and trust—specifically, our trust in the external world. It can also relate to financial security and physical safety.

Signature shapes: Increased curvature (lordosis) or a flattening of the lower back (loss of natural curve).

Spinal archetypes: The Lone Wolf and the Dependent.

The Lone Wolf (The Flattening)

A flat lower back (loss of the natural curve) falls into the archetype of the hyper-independent. The person who says, "I'll just do it myself." They rarely ask for help and often learned that they could not rely on others—perhaps they were let down or had to grow up too fast—and the body braced itself. This flattening is a physical manifestation of a lack of trust in the support of the universe or other people. A person with a flattening of the lumbar spine carries the weight of the world and often has a core belief that no one will catch them if they fall.

The Dependent (Increased Curve)

An exaggerated sway in the lower back (hyper-lordosis) often signals the opposite of the lone wolf—an increased need for dependence. The person with this signature trait may feel like they cannot do it alone. They may feel ungrounded, overwhelmed by life's responsibilities, and constantly seeking assistance or reassurance. The deep sway is almost an energetic collapse, a physical plea for support because the internal foundation of the solar plexus feels insufficient to hold them upright.

The Upper Back (Thoracic)

Structure: The thoracic spine consists of 12 vertebrae (T1–T12) that provide structural stability and protect vital organs such as our heart and lungs. The thoracic spine enables rotation and movement while protecting the spinal cord. It runs from the base of the neck down to the abdomen and is the only spinal region attached to the rib cage.

Energetic center: The upper and mid-back houses the energy center of your heart and is aligned with the heart chakra.

Relational language: The state of our upper back tells the story of how we relate to love, connection, and self-worth.

Signature shapes: Increased curvature of the upper back or hunch known as a kyphotic curve, or the inverse of a flattening.

Spinal archetypes: The Hunch and the Shield.

The Hunch (Kyphotic Curve)

When we see an exaggerated outward curvature in the upper back (kyphosis)—a rounding of the shoulders that closes off the chest—we are looking at a pattern of protection. Energetically, this archetype is often linked to an anxious attachment style. People who have this curve might crave connection and security but fundamentally lack confidence in their own worthiness. They "armor" their heart to protect it from rejection or pain. They may feel a void inside that they are trying to fill through others, latching onto relationships or external validation to feel safe. The hunch is the body's way of curling in on itself, shielding the most vulnerable part of the emotional anatomy: the heart.

The Shield (Flattening)

Conversely, there is the flattening of the thoracic spine—where the natural curve is rigid and straight—and this is often the avoidant archetype. They might be disconnected from their heart center, hypovigilant, emotionally unavailable, or cut off from their own feelings. Where the hunched person is desperately seeking connection, the flattened person is often pushing it away to maintain control. They have learned that it is safer not to feel, and their spine has rigidified to ensure that the "messiness" of emotion doesn't get in. They are often hyper-independent, not because they want to be, but because they learned they had to be.

The Neck (Cervical)

Structure: The neck is built of seven stacked bones (C1–C7). The cervical spine is a highly flexible, lordotic-curved structure that supports the head, protects the spinal cord, and enables movement and rotation.

Energetic center: The neck is the bridge between the head and the heart. It houses the throat chakra and connects to the higher centers of intuition (Third Eye) and connection (Crown).

Relational language: The state of the neck tells the story of how we relate to expression and our own mind and intuition.

Signature shapes: Upper neck and mid-neck tension and pain.

Spinal archetypes: The Overachiever and the Metamorphosis.

The Overachiever (Upper Neck Tension)

Neck pain is perhaps the most common symptom we see in the West, and it is almost always linked to the Type A personality. We see this pattern constantly in high-performers. There is immense tension at the very top of the neck (the occiput) and these archetypes are "wired but tired"—unable to switch off the monkey mind. They need background noise to relax because silence is too confronting. They might resonate with living life entirely in their head, meaning they are constantly analyzing, strategizing, and striving.

They might feel disconnected from their heart and body because they are too busy trying to achieve self-worth through external accomplishments. They are focused on tasks and keeping themselves busy rather than just being.

The Metamorphosis (Mid-Neck Tension)

Tension in the middle of the neck often relates to the throat chakra—the center of truth and expression. These are the people who have spent their entire lives living for everyone else. They have repressed their voice to keep the peace, or perhaps they swing to the other extreme of over-sharing without boundaries.

Chronic tension here tells us a story of repression: *What have you swallowed? What truth are you not speaking? Or, conversely, are you speaking too much without thinking and creating conflict that isn't aligned with your soul?*

When I see this pattern, it often signals that they are in a "metamorphosis" phase. They are starting to ask the big questions: *Who am I? What is my legacy? What do I actually want?* They are shedding an old skin. The tension in the neck is the friction between the person they were told to be and the person they are becoming.

The Sacrum

Structure: The sacrum is the triangular-shaped bone at the base of the spine, made up of a group of five fused vertebrae (S1–S5).

Energetic center: The sacrum acts as a sacred anchoring point to the inner self, linking the upper and lower body. It's associated with the sacral chakra and the root chakra.

Relational language: The sacrum acts like your internal compass and is considered a "sacred bone." It's the seat of Kundalini energy and intimate connection with yourself, sexuality, and emotions.

Signature shapes: Tension in the sacrum or imbalance between the lower and upper spinal centers.

Spinal archetypes: The Pleaser and the Boiling Pot.

The Pleaser

At the start of a course, I often ask my students, "How many of you had to ask someone else's permission or opinion before you signed up for this course?" The ones who raise their hands usually have tension in their sacrum. This area gets blocked when we outsource our intuition. It is the archetype of the person who knows the answer but is terrified to act on it without validation. They leak energy thinking about "what ifs" and "should haves," paralyzed by a lack of self-trust. They obsess over possibilities and seek confirmation from the outside world. The disconnection creates a feeling of being unmoored, unable to rest in the certainty of their own innate wisdom.

The Boiling Pot

There is also an archetype that has a fear-loop pattern between the coccyx and occiput. This is a pattern where there is intense tension at the very bottom of the spine (the tailbone/coccyx) and the very top of the spine (the neck) or base of the skull (occiput).

This is the archetype of high anxiety.

The tension at both ends of the spine creates a taut wire of fear. This is not the depression of the past; this is the anxiety of the future. They feel like a pot of water on the stove that is about to boil over. Their capacity for stress is maxed out; it takes only the slightest trigger to make them react. They are ungrounded (coccyx tension) and overthinking (neck tension), leaving them hovering in a state of hypervigilance and disconnected from the safety of the present moment.

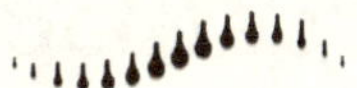

These symptoms are not random. When you bend over to pick up a pen and your back seizes, it isn't because the pen was too heavy. It is because your system was already carrying a thousand pounds of emotional weight and the pen was what finally tipped the scales over.

The spine expresses what the mind represses.

CHAPTER 6

Working With Spinal Archetypes

The first rule of Spinal Energetics is that these patterns are not inherently "bad," nor are they something that needs to be "fixed" in the traditional sense. They are protective strategies created by your innate intelligence to help you survive difficult moments in your life.

They serve a purpose. The problem only arises when you have outgrown the need for the armor, but the body hasn't received the memo.

The Illusion of Safety

When we look at these archetypes, we are often looking at a nervous system frozen in fear. Usually, the client's "worst-case scenario" has actually come true in the past, so they live with a heightened sense of fear that something to the same extreme will happen again.

This is why simple reassurance doesn't work. You can tell a client, "You're safe now," but if their body is stuck in a trauma loop, those words are empty.

I also want to address a dangerous misconception I see in the spiritual community. I have had clients tell me that previous teachers told them they "attracted" their trauma—that there was something in their energetic field that drew in an abusive partner, a medical condition, or a horrific event, for example.

I want to be very clear: this is victim-blaming disguised as empowerment. I do not believe it is in anyone's dharma to have bad things happen to them. Sometimes people do bad things because they are unwell and accidents simply happen. Telling a survivor they are responsible for their trauma might seem like it helps them feel in control of their future, but in reality, it is incredibly disempowering and keeps them trapped in self-doubt.

Our goal is not to blame the client, but to help them find contextual safety. We want to move the nervous system from a generalized fear ("All men are a threat") to a contextual truth ("That specific man was a threat, but I am safe with this man now"). We help the body sort through what is a real, present-time reaction and what is an old pattern playing out.

The Archetype Assessment

So, how do we determine which archetype is active?

Like a traditional chiropractor or physician, we start by assessing the physical body to see where in the spine the issue is manifesting. We compare leg length, as discrepancies show which side of the body holds the tension pattern, and we also look at the Achilles tendon, as it's actually like a miniature spine and can give us clues about where to look in the actual spine. Once we have completed this assessment, we then delve into the energetic layers on the physical spine, which is what we refer to as the "major spine" or "real spine."

We check the level of life force and innate intelligence coming through this point by placing our fingers there and observing how the body responds—the body will show you what kind of connection it has. It might move in a way that reveals it's welcoming and fluid, or it might have a tension or stiffness to it that shows there's trauma in that.

Body responses all indicate a story. But it's important to remember that when we first start looking into what's happening, what shows up to us first may not be the priority or the full story. It's rare that people come in as open books, fully trusting the practitioner to delve into their deepest inner workings. Some might consciously think they are, yet their bodies will subconsciously protect their hearts, for example. There might be another section in the spine that must be looked at first in order to get to the true area of need.

That happens a lot. For example, with the thoracic, which is the heart's energetic center, a lot of people aren't ready for you to go straight in as it's a very large protective strategy. They'll show you other layers until they can open up that deeper layer. So for the first few sessions, it's usually more surface level until we can build trust with the body and get deeper. It's only with trust that we can find the true source of the pain or tension.

When you place your fingers on an area of the spine you may notice…

Flexible and fluid body movements and strong life force =
an openness to development and personal insight.

A tight and locked body with low vitality =
someone who is under stress and in protective mode.

Once we have assessed the level of tension and life force coming through there, then we would move onto what we call the energetic spines. These are located in different parts of the body but they refer back to points on the spine. It's similar to reflexology in this way, where different points in our hands and feet relate to different body parts. We do the same check that we did on the physical spine, examining what the inner intelligence is communicating to us here.

What we are looking for is the point of disconnection between the two and finding the innate knowing that is holding onto this protective strategy. We're trying to connect to that inner wisdom so then it can unwind itself and remember who it truly is.

Remember: every protective strategy or tension pattern in the body holds the same intelligence that created it in the first place. All we're doing as a practitioner is trying to connect to that, and we do this by searching through the layers and finding where the root is. So we might start with the physical layer, and if there's no connection or resonance, then we know it's not a physical issue and we move on to the next layer until we find what we're looking for.

It's a system and process you can trust, as the body reveals things to you and shows you where to look.

The Five Energetic Layers

- **Physical:** A physical, structural injury or tension.
- **Emotional:** Unprocessed and suppressed emotions that become stuck.
- **Mental:** A story that has been created and perpetuated, keeping them stuck and in a loop (a limiting belief, for example).
- **Spiritual (Surrogation):** An empathetic load of sorts, perhaps carrying a burden, trauma or emotion for someone else, like a partner or parent.
- **Personal Soul:** The authentic self—a disconnect between what their soul needs and what their reality is or a lesson that is connected to essential growth.

Once we find the layer where the resonance lives, we act almost like a virus scanner on a computer. We gently point it out: "Hey, the virus is here. You put it here for a reason. Do you remember?" And the inner intelligence responds, "Oh, yes I do remember. That's right. I remember why I've done this, but I recognize that in this present moment, in this safety that I have right now, I no longer need to hold onto this."

That's why it's really important for the practitioner to create a safe environment where fear cannot exist, because the soul and the spine won't release if there is any fear or judgment present.

When we make this connection, the body starts to physically "unwind" and find its way back to itself. So that's the movement we see when people get Spinal Energetics done. They move independently of their mind as their spines and bodies unwind the tension and protective strategy. It's about getting back to yourself and realizing that you are not a prisoner to what has happened to you—you can live freely based on the safety of the present, rather than the survival of the past. However, this work isn't about erasing your past—you wouldn't want to lose the wisdom of your experiences—but it's about changing your perception of them so you are no longer chained to them. We are moving you from a state of reaction (living in the past trauma) to a state of creation (living in the present potential).

Caitlin's Case Study

Caitlin was a woman in her early 40s who had lived with a persistent tightness through the middle of her spine for years. She described it as if her body was "always bracing for something." There was nothing she could think of that had happened recently to cause this, yet her nervous system behaved as though a threat was always nearby waiting. She'd tried many different approaches like exercise, physio and massage therapy, but the tension would temporarily ease and then just return again.

When she first came in, it was as if the body was guarded. Her breathing was shallow and the thoracic spine held a subtle rigidity, as though the muscles had learned to constantly remain on standby. This is something I see often and it is the body holding a protective strategy long after the original moment that required it has passed.

During the session, we located the layer where the resonance of that tension seemed to live. Not the muscles themselves, but the pattern beneath them—the protective intelligence that had once helped the body survive a difficult experience years earlier.

When the nervous system senses safety, it begins to reveal these patterns. Slowly, her spine began to move in small, involuntary waves. Her shoulders rolled slightly, then her rib cage expanded and contracted as though the body was rediscovering how to breathe freely again. The movements were not directed by her thinking mind—they were the body's way of unwinding a strategy that had been held for a very long time.

Afterward, she described a simple but profound realization: the tension she had carried for so many years no longer felt necessary. The body seemed to recognize that the conditions that once required protection were no longer present.

What changed was not the past (those experiences shaped her and remained part of her life story), but the body no longer needed to organize itself around them.

This is the shift I often describe to clients. The nervous system can live in a state of reaction, continually responding to what has already happened, or it can move into a state of creation, where the body begins organizing itself around the safety and possibility of the present moment.

When that shift occurs, the spine and the person begin to move differently through the world.

As we move forward into the deeper mechanics of this work, carry this knowledge with you:

Your spine is
not just a stack
of bones. It is a
spiritual highway.
It is the story of
your life.
And no matter
how twisted or
tense the plot has
become, there is
always a way
back to the truth
of who you are.

The Spine Holds Your Story:
A Map of Spinal Energetics

Spinal Archetypes:
The Language of Your Posture

The Neck (Cervical): The Bridge of Expression

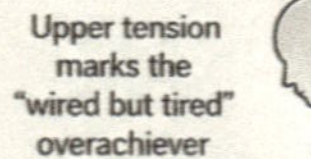
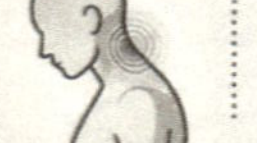

Upper tension marks the "wired but tired" overachiever while mid-neck tension signals a soul-level metamorphosis.

Relational Language: Truth, Expression, & Intuition

The Upper Back (Thoracic): The Heart's Armor

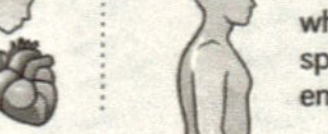

A hunch (kyphosis) shields the heart from rejection while a rigid, flat spine indicates emotional avoidance.

Relational Language: Love, Connection, & Self-Worth

The Lower Back (Lumbar): The Foundation

Reflects survival and trust; a flat back indicates hyper-independence while an increased curve suggests a plea for support.

Relational Language: Safety, Survival, & Trust

The Sacrum: The Internal Compass

Acts as the sacred bone and seat of intimate connection with yourself, sexuality and emotions.

Tension in the sacrum reflects an imbalance between the lower and upper spinal centers.

Relational Language: Intimacy, Desire, & Sovereignty

The Path to Unwinding

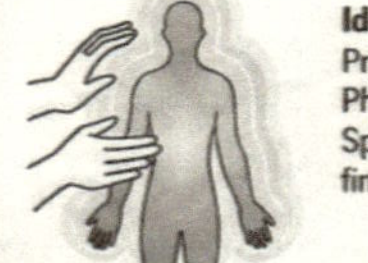

Identify the Layer of Resonance: Practitioners scan five layers—Physical, Mental, Emotional, Spiritual, and Personal Soul—to find where the story lives.

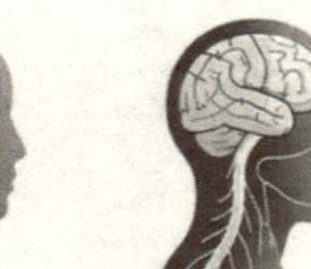

From Reaction to Creation: Healing involves moving the nervous system from past survival patterns into present-moment safety and potential.

> "The body expresses what the mind represses."

Posture is a direct reflection of how a person is currently functioning in life.

CHAPTER 7

The Shape Between Who You Were and Who You Are

Healing through the spine is not about fixing a "bad" back. It is about recognizing that the shape you are in—your posture, your tension, your pain—is a protective strategy. Your body didn't twist or tighten to hurt you; it did it to keep you safe.

The pain arises when those old shapes no longer fit the person you are becoming. It is the friction between your survival self and your authentic self.

Going back to the client who suffered from chronic bronchitis, there was a massive misalignment between who she was and the version of her that was able to show up at work. She was in an environment where she was unheard and repressed, so her body created an inflammation in her throat and lungs. When she removed herself from that environment, the "cure" came in the form of alignment.

This is the core of Spinal Energetics: closing the gap between your soul and your reality.

We live in a society that encourages this gap. We are taught to chase whichever version of success is trending at the time and strive for the things that look good on paper, even if they feel empty in our souls. We compete with people we don't know to impress people we don't like. And the bigger the gap between your soul's truth and your daily reality, the more pain you will have in your spine.

I see this difference starkly when I travel. In the East—in places like India or the Philippines—the spinal issues are different. They have physical deformities from carrying heavy loads or malnutrition, but they don't have the same psycho-emotional tension patterns we see in the West. They don't have the "hamster wheel" tension in the lower back. Their life is harder physically, but often simpler spiritually. There is less friction between who they are and who they think they should be. They have a level of acceptance and community that buffers the stress.

In the West, we have everything, yet we are burnt out, anxious and in pain. We have "options fatigue"—like going to a nail salon and being overwhelmed by 70 colors or a restaurant with a four-page menu. We think freedom is having endless choice, but true freedom is knowing yourself so well that the choice is obvious.

I learned this through my own life. I never wanted to be a divorced person. I came from a broken home, and I wanted the happy ending. I was with my husband for 14 years, and he was (and is) a beautiful man. He did nothing wrong. But my soul started speaking to me. Every morning and every night, a voice would say: *This isn't for you anymore.*

I'd wake up and I'd hear, *This isn't for you anymore.* Every night before I went to sleep: *This isn't for you anymore…* I meditated and it kept saying it. *It's not for you.* It was the opposite of what I wanted and I was getting angry at my soul. I was like, *Can you just shut up? I don't want to leave. I'm happy.*

I fought it. I got angry at it. I wanted to stay in the safety of the known. But the voice was relentless. It wasn't a voice of fear—fear is frantic and loud. This was a soul voice: quiet, repetitive, and unyielding.

Leaving was the hardest thing I ever did. It shattered the picture of what my life was supposed to be. But the moment I left, the voice stopped. I haven't heard it since.

It was almost like a fight between my soul and myself because on my earthly level, I said I'd marry this person. I said I'd be with them forever. My values around my humanness and society were at war with my soul. I never wanted to be a divorced person or someone who "gives" up. My mum had come from divorce, so that was something I never wanted.

And my husband hadn't done anything wrong either. Most people are like, "Oh, why'd you split up? Did he have an affair? Did you cheat? Was he a gambler? Like what happened?"

I reply to people's questions with, "Nothing, my soul just kept telling me that it wasn't for me anymore." It's not a common explanation. And while sometimes I struggle with the divorce, I don't struggle with my heart because I don't look at it as a failure. I was with someone I love for 14 years. We're still friends and we're still respectful of each other, which I think is true unconditional love.

I still can't tell you why my soul said that, but I've never heard the voice say, "You shouldn't have done that."

I think we often make mistakes in believing that the soul's messages are only going to be for what will make us happiest at that point in time. But really it's planning for our *true* happiness—the one where we know we are completely aligned.

Spinal Energetics didn't exist until I left that marriage. If I had stayed in the "safety" of the misalignment, I would never have birthed this work.

As hard as it is to action sometimes, I just can't live my life not connected to that voice. So whatever that guides me to do, I do. Whether it's what I want or what I don't want, because I trust its guidance and living life without its guidance is not peaceful. I don't need an easy life, because my life was actually easier before and it's not even that I'm happier as such, like I didn't just leave and become purely happy. But I became more peaceful and more myself, and there's a happiness that comes with that. It's a deeper happiness, not a happiness manufactured by the matrix.

There is a price to pay for living authentically. You might disappoint people. You might have less money for a while. You might lose the status of being a "good wife" or a "corporate success." But there is a bigger price to pay for living inauthentically. That price is paid in your body. It is paid in autoimmune diseases, in depression, in chronic fatigue, and in a spine that twists to accommodate a life that doesn't fit you.

"I speak two languages, Body and English."
Mae West

Love Is the Alignment Your Spine Is Looking For

I recently watched the Netflix documentary *Street Food: Asia*, which features the legendary Jay Fai (Supinya Junsuta), the 81-year-old Bangkok street food chef covered in her episode *Jay Fai: Fire & Soul.*

Born around 1945 to Chinese immigrant parents, Jay Fai grew up in a poor neighborhood in Bangkok where her family sold chicken noodles. Since she wasn't a confident cook, she chose a different path and became a seamstress. However, when a fire destroyed her tailoring shop in her 30s, she returned to the family food business to survive.

While learning to cook, she accidentally discovered her signature technique. One night she overheated her wok and rather than waste the ingredients, she threw the noodles into the blazing pan. The intense heat and minimal oil created a delicious smoky, charred flavor that would become known as "wok hei."

Today, Jay Fai cooks every dish herself over charcoal, famously wearing ski goggles to protect her eyes from the heat and smoke. Despite being a street-side stall, her restaurant Raan Jay Fai uses premium ingredients like large mud crab in dishes such as her famous crab omelet and drunken noodles.

In 2018, her small open-air restaurant earned one Michelin star in the first Bangkok Michelin Guide, making her the only street food vendor with that distinction at the time. She is still the sole cook at her restaurant and works countless hours. She hasn't had a day off in 40 years and yet she's not burnt out. She was still talking about it as if she was just as passionate as the first day.

And so what's the difference? How are most of us so burnt out?

Firstly, Jay's work has meaning for her. It had connection to her family and alignment to her soul. She is overjoyed to serve others with her passion. She sees cooking as part of her destiny. The second difference is that she says the secret ingredients are love and heart.

When you're doing something with love in the world, it won't burn you out.

The Spine Adjusts Itself

Spinal Energetics is about peeling back the layers of conditioning—the "shoulds," the "musts," the fear of judgment. To walk your dharma and discover what makes you feel like you, what makes you come alive and what makes you feel aligned with love.

Spinal Energetics is listening to that deeper voice and giving it space to find its home.

This process isn't always blissful. Real healing is not just lying on a table and floating away into the cosmos. Sometimes it means confronting the fact that you hate your job, realizing your relationship is over, or feeling the grief of a parent who is still alive but no longer present—like my own experience with my mother.

The movements you see on the Spinal Energetics table—the shaking, the arching, the unwinding—this is the body processing that gap. It is the nervous system discharging the energy of the "false self" to make room for the "true self." It is like how animals shake off trauma in the wild. We have forgotten how to do this because we are too busy holding it together. We are too busy being polite. Too busy dancing to society's beat and forgetting the rhythm in our own heart.

When you allow your spine to unwind, you are not just releasing tension; you are recovering your intuition. You are polishing the compass. You are moving from a life of "toxic success" to a life of soul alignment. And when you are in alignment, you don't need to be perfect. You don't need to be happy all the time. You just need to be real.

Your body is your greatest ally.
It is the one thing that will never lie to you.

Why Modern Medicine Misses the Pain Origin

If the spine is so clearly communicating, why does modern medicine so often fail to hear it? The answer lies in our fundamental model of health. We have built a system that views the body as a machine. If a car breaks down, you take it to a mechanic to replace the part. We treat the body with the same philosophy: "Pain equals problem, fix problem, pain goes away." But we are not cars. We are complex, multidimensional human beings.

Brigitta's Case Study

I had a client Brigitta who came to me as a last resort. She was 39 and was suffering from debilitating neck pain that radiated down into both her arms. Because of her age and wellness lifestyle, her pain didn't make sense as there was no obvious explanation. She had already been treated by an osteopath, physiotherapist and chiropractor, but there had been no improvement. She was convinced that something was dreadfully wrong, so she asked for an MRI. The results? Clean. There was a little bit of degeneration, but it was in the normal range for her age. Her spine health appeared to be well, yet she was in severe pain. The X-ray is often able to suggest the symptomology within the person, but not with Brigitta.

The medical professionals told her there was

"nothing really wrong." They implied she was healthy, but her pain said otherwise. This is where the modern medical model hits its limits: if the machine can't see it, it must not exist. Or worse, it's psychogenic—a polite way of saying it's all in your head. But pain generated by emotional distress lights up the exact same pain centers in the brain as pain generated by a broken bone.[49] To the brain, the pain is identical.

When I assessed Brigitta, there was a little bit of rotation in her hip but nothing too bad. Normally, when the hips are out of alignment, it increases the pressure in the neck. Even from a traditional sense, if you release the piriformis muscle or the glute muscle, it can release tension in the neck even without touching the neck physically.

When I felt Brigitta's neck, there was a little bit of inflammation. The pain she was feeling was similar and just as real as someone with a disc issue or serious neck issue. It's very difficult for clients with this type of pain, as they feel like they're going crazy because they're always being told there's no reason for it. But it's not true. It's just that there's no physical reason in the eyes of traditional healthcare.

I moved down her spine and I felt a huge amount of tension in her nervous system, right near her bra line. That's a sign of a nervous system locked in a sympathetic, fight-or-flight state. The point representing her vagus nerve was also tender and tight, meaning she had no access to rest or digest. That means the vagus nerve is working too hard and she's not getting into a parasympathetic state, which requires rest and sleep. The inflammation on the back of her neck was coming more from an emotional aspect, and you can tell because physical inflammation looks and feels different from emotional. The physical layer is a little bit harder to push, whereas the emotional inflammation feels softer to push. Chemical stress feels different as well—it's squishier. In this client's instance, her neck was inflamed with emotions.

So we did Spinal Energetics and a gentle process in her emotional field across her spine, in the neck and also in her pelvis. And she felt a lot of relief. It turned out she was carrying immense grief from a pregnancy loss and unvoiced issues in her relationship. Her body wasn't wrong in communicating this pain, it just wasn't being understood by practitioners who were looking for a physical cause when it was actually a problem designed by her innate intelligence to force her to look at an emotional one. If you are not able to feel the emotion that's in you, the body will find another way to get you to connect to it. And so the body's like, *Hey, you're not doing the emotional work, you're not looking at this aspect, so we are going to create a physical problem.* So that actually makes you stop and makes you pay attention to it because you weren't paying attention to it before.

This is where modern medicine fails people. We treat the physical symptom and ignore the metaphysical cause. To me, what she came in with was pretty textbook. But she'd seen other practitioners who'd made her feel like she was crazy. She heard gaslighting statements such as: "You're healthy," or "You're being a hypochondriac." Her anxiety levels peaked and perpetuated her nervous system into a vicious cycle of stress. Often, someone's anxiety and stress increase the pain and it becomes a loop that can be very challenging to get out of.

Disorders and *Dis-order*

Clients often come in with chronic bloating or IBS, unable to find relief even though they've been on every FODMAP diet and taken every probiotic. But the gut is connected to the brain via the vagus nerve, so if you are living in a state of chronic stress, your vagus nerve is constantly overstimulated and it shuts down your digestion. The problem isn't the food; it's the nervous system. You can't diet your way out of nervous system dysregulation.

We also see this connection with fibromyalgia—a chronic pain disorder that is usually from trauma manifesting in sensations of body pain years later. The medical treatment for fibromyalgia is often antidepressants (SSRIs) or anti-anxiety medication, which helps manage the symptoms. By prescribing this, the medical system is admitting that the root cause is mental and emotional, yet they treat it with a chemical band-aid rather than helping the person integrate the trauma stored in their body.

This happens across the board. If something happens, like an assault or other traumatic event, we are advised to see a psychiatrist or a psychologist as the main form of healing. While talk therapy and cognitive behavioral therapy are very useful, there are studies that show people find talking about what happened to them retraumatizing. The body can't tell the difference between reality and imagination. So even though they're just talking about the event, their body is affected and feels a physiological response as if that was happening again.

This also links back to what we asserted in an earlier chapter about how the brain can shut down in the area that governs talking when reliving the trauma, which essentially suppresses the event and stops them from fully processing it. So talk therapy can work with the mental processing to an extent, but it's not working with the body and the way it stores its own information. It comes back to the conscious versus unconscious. Rationally we understand that "Okay, this happened, and I want to move forward, I want to let go of this." But wanting to let go of something and actually embodying the feeling of letting go are two very different things. With Spinal Energetics, the hope is to embody that feeling of letting go as opposed to just knowing that you need to let go to move on.

Eating disorders are another condition where the psyche is connected to the body. It used to be treated purely as a dietetic issue, and patients would go in and have feeding tubes inserted to make them put on weight. They would be educated by a dietitian on what and how to eat. But they missed out on the *why*. We've changed now, as they've realized treating the physical symptoms are not enough. It's not the education of what to eat, it's about figuring out what part of them doesn't want to eat. What part of them believes they don't even deserve food. There's something going on emotionally, and Spinal Energetics can help them understand it.

These people have found Spinal Energetics so helpful because it was getting them connected back to their body, which is something that they'd been frightened to be connected to for so long. It also allowed them to get to the deeper meaning as to why they were using food, because it's never really about the food, as their way of coping in the world. Whether that's overeating or undereating, it's either to numb something because they don't want to feel it or to give them a sense of control they lost at some point in their life. It's never just the food, and the same thing goes for substance abuse.

These things are all emotionally instigated responses. And that's why they're quite difficult for us to heal in a system that looks only to the physical.

In cases of chronic pain with an emotional causation, it can be difficult to resolve because the person often needs to address their environment. Often, it means making a change in their life and in the relationships with themselves and others.

So, if you assess someone's symptoms from a purely physical point of view and not look deeper, that person is going to go back into the same environment and encounter the same original stresses. And therefore, the back pain, neck pain or other symptoms will only have a short-term resolution before reappearing again. The reason it's coming back all the time is because the metaphysical within the environment hasn't been addressed.

Looking at the whole person allows the body to rest in a safe space and be seen in all aspects. And I think that's where, for a lack of better word, the shortcut is. Spinal Energetics connects them to their truth. It turns down the volume on the excess noise and turns up the volume on their innate intelligence. It prioritizes what needs to be looked at so that you can remember who you really are and what's important to your soul.

An important distinction to make is that we're not trying to fix anyone. Although my goal is to relieve the physical pain, I don't relieve them of the actual pain. Instead, I connect to the part of them that is asking for them to make the connection and to relieve it themselves.

If we cover the pain with bucketloads of medication and painkillers, we cannot fully hear what the body is signaling. And it always has something important to say.

"Our bodies are apt to be our autobiographies."

FRANK GILLETTE BURGESS

PART THREE

THE STORY YOU'RE CARRYING

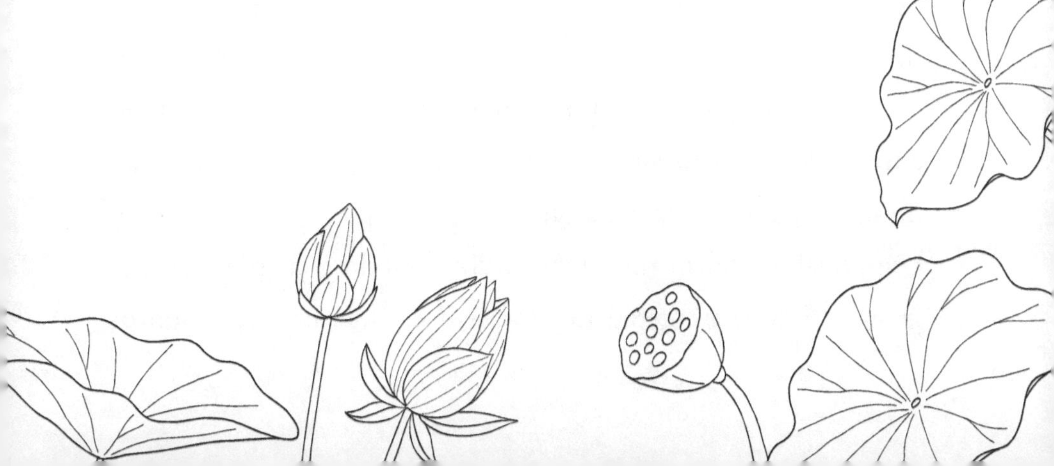

Your spine is a living, breathing holograph of every experience you've ever had—both the ones you remember and, perhaps more importantly, the ones you have tried to forget. In the world of Spinal Energetics, we don't just see a "herniated disc" or "tight traps"; we see the physical remnants of a child who had to grow up too fast, a professional who sacrificed their dream for a title and financial security, or a partner who has been carrying the weight of a dying marriage for a decade.

However, the story goes much deeper than your own timeline.

When we are born, we are not a "clean slate," as philosopher John Locke theorized in the 17th century. Locke argued that we are born without innate ideas, and that all knowledge comes from experience, and while he wasn't entirely wrong, the theory of "Nature versus Nurture" has evolved significantly. We now know that the "slate" comes to us with some text already written on it.

As we discussed earlier regarding the work of Dr. Bruce Lipton, our DNA is not a fixed, unchangeable blueprint that dictates our destiny. Instead, it is a library of possibilities. Our experiences—and the environments we inhabit—determine which "books" are taken off the shelf and read. A clear example of this is schizophrenia. Modern psychiatry views this through the "Diathesis-Stress Model," which suggests that while a person may carry a genetic predisposition for the disorder, it may remain entirely dormant throughout their life. It is only when the environment provides a specific, high-intensity "input"—such as severe emotional trauma or the chemical shock of drug abuse—that the genetic code is triggered to express itself. The manifestation of the disorder only occurs when the stress on the system exceeds its capacity to remain in balance. This means that the stories we carry often begin long before our first breath.

This is because the experiences of our parents, grandparents, and even our great-grandparents are passed down to us through intergenerational trauma. Science shows us that trauma can leave a chemical mark on our genes, altering how our nervous system responds to stress. You might carry a baseline level of anxiety that doesn't belong to you. It may be the "energetic echo" of a grandmother who lived through a war or a father who never felt safe in his own home. Your spine, as the primary highway of the nervous system, archives these ancestral echoes, holding them in its curves and tensions to keep you "prepared" for a danger you've never personally met.

On top of this ancestral foundation, we layer our own unique experiences. Every interaction, every belief, and every opinion we hold about ourselves and the world acts as a fresh stroke of the pen. Even seemingly meaningless conversations either confirm or deny our internal narrative, contributing to the story we tell ourselves about who we are and what is possible.

In the simplest of terms, our brains and nervous systems are like a highly sophisticated computer.

- **DNA is the software** created by the manufacturer, loaded with ancestral data.
- **Our experiences are the code** input by the "engineer" of our lives.
- **Our bodies and beliefs are the printouts.**

When we are in pain, it is often because of a "print error." There is a smudge on an important line of code, or the output looks vastly different from how it displays on the screen. This is a disconnect. To find out what that disconnect is, we must look at both the inherited software and the code we have written ourselves through our habits, roles, and reactions.

To heal what our spines are communicating, we must first learn to read the story. We must understand how these narratives became calcified into our posture and how our innate intelligence has been using pain as a messenger to get us back into alignment.

CHAPTER 8

INTERGENERATIONAL TRAUMA

Intergenerational trauma is the transmission of the effects of trauma from one generation to the next. From a neuroscience perspective, this functions via a fascinating and complex bridge between the brain's architecture and our chemical gene expression.

When a person experiences significant trauma—be it one big event or the chronic little stressors of systemic oppression or poverty—their brain literally rewires itself to ensure survival. The amygdala (the brain's alarm system) becomes hyper-reactive, while the prefrontal cortex (the seat of logic and regulation) may become underactive. Additionally, the Hypothalamic-Pituitary-Adrenal (HPA) axis—the system that governs our stress response—gets "stuck" in a state of high alert.[50]

Through epigenetics, these changes don't always stop with the individual. Trauma can leave chemical "tags" (known as methyl groups) on our DNA.[51] These tags don't change the DNA sequence itself, but they act like a dimmer switch, turning certain genes up or down. If your mother lived in a state of chronic PTSD, her body may have passed down a "pre-set" HPA axis to you. You didn't inherit her memories, but you inherited her stress physiology. You were born with a nervous system already braced for a world that it perceives as inherently unsafe.

Let's look at how this manifests physically in the spine, specifically within the lower back region.

Imagine a woman whose grandmother lived through a period of extreme displacement and poverty—perhaps a refugee experience where safety and home were never guaranteed. That grandmother's nervous system would have lived in a state of perpetual survival, likely manifesting in a physical bracing of the lower back and pelvis—the areas associated with our foundational security and belonging.

Her DNA carries the "code" for this survival strategy. Two generations later, her granddaughter—who lives in a comfortable suburb in Melbourne and has never known true scarcity—struggles with chronic, idiopathic lower back pain and a pervasive sense of anxiety about her financial security.

On an X-ray, the granddaughter's spine might show a flat back or significant tension in the psoas muscle. Physically, she hasn't done anything to cause this pain. However, she is carrying the ancestral story. Her innate intelligence is still running the "Survival in Scarcity" software that was necessary for her grandmother but is now a print error in her modern life. Her spine is literally braced against a famine that isn't happening.

The Compounding Epigenetic Load

This brings us to a vital question: why are we seeing such a massive spike in mental health disorders and chronic pain today?

While better diagnostics and reduced stigma play a role, we must also consider the compounding epigenetic load. Each generation is *not* starting from zero. We are starting with the accumulated, unintegrated baggage of the 18th, 19th, and 20th centuries—centuries defined by world wars, industrialization, and rapid societal upheaval.

Intergenerational trauma has been clinically recognized since the 1960s. It was first observed in the children of Holocaust survivors.[52] Clinicians noticed that trauma-related symptoms were present in individuals even when they had grown up in security and safety and without any direct exposure to violence or threat to their care. Yet their nervous systems inherited patterns of hypervigilance, emotional dysregulation, or dissociation, without knowing why. Psychiatrist Bessel van der Kolk, author of *The Body Keeps the Score,* suggests that trauma is stored in the body and nervous system, not solely in conscious memory.[53] Trauma returns to us as a reaction, not a memory. The inability to access a conscious story can deepen the individual's confusion and shame. *Nothing bad happened to me, so why do I feel this way? Why do I react this way?*

Think of each generation as adding a new layer of code to the software.

If a grandfather lived through the trauma of war and never integrated that experience, his nervous system remained in a state of high alert. Through epigenetics and unconscious body memory, that state of hypervigilance is passed down—not as a memory of the war itself, but as a **biological predisposition** to anxiety.

If the next generation then experiences their own unique stressors—perhaps modern corporate burnout or a broken marriage—they are adding their own trauma on top of an already sensitized foundation.

We aren't just starting from scratch; we are starting with a nervous system that is already pre-tuned to a frequency of survival rather than safety.

The software is trying to protect us from a threat that is no longer there, leading to a massive disconnect. This is why sometimes we encounter a small stress and the effect is not equal to the cause. **The system is simply at capacity.**

We are carrying the ghosts of our lineage in our marrow, and our spines are buckling under the weight of a narrative that is becoming increasingly complex and "noisy," as each generation is inheriting a slightly more burdened vessel.

When a client walks into a Spinal Energetics session today, we aren't just working with their 30 or 40 years of life; we are potentially working with a century of braced nervous systems.

Unintegrated Trauma Echoes

The second way our code is fundamentally created is through our environment in our early years (usually up to six years of age). As children, our nervous systems are essentially co-regulated by our parents. We are like mirrors, reflecting the energetic state of our caregivers long before we have the cognitive ability to understand their words. More than that though, we also model and integrate their behaviors, thoughts, opinions and beliefs.

If a parent is operating from a place of unintegrated trauma, they are subconsciously passing that same trauma onto the child through their behavior. They may be physically present but energetically checked out, or perhaps they are hyper-vigilant and controlling. They might believe that they are not good enough, are not worthy of love or that bad things will always happen to them. There's a good chance that these will be passed onto the child as well and they won't remember ever living without them.

As a child, you absorb this as the default setting for what life is.

- You learn that to be safe, you must be quiet (cervical/neck tension).
- You learn that to be loved, you must be perfect (thoracic/heart bracing).
- You learn that the world is dangerous, so you must be strong (lumbar/sacral rigidity).

You haven't experienced the original trauma, but you have absorbed the aftereffects so deeply that they become your own belief system. You are essentially living in a house built from someone else's blueprints, wondering why the hallways feel too narrow for your soul.

Emma's Case Study

Emma came in with persistent lower back pain and a deep pelvic "holding" pattern that hadn't responded to physical treatment. She had tried bodywork, myotherapy and physiotherapy, but nothing seemed to relieve the feeling of holding tension.

What stood out wasn't just the location of the pain, but the quality of it. It wasn't sharp or reactive like an acute case; it was constant and she described it as feeling contained and "almost deliberate." As though her body was holding something in place.

When I worked with her spine, the lower segments didn't behave like a typical mechanical issue that we see in the lower back. There was very little variability and the area stayed organized in the same protective pattern—even when the rest of the system began to shift.

That kind of consistency is something I pay attention to because it often suggests that the body isn't responding to the present moment alone, but to something more ingrained.

As we spoke, there was a clear family history of women who had endured loss, emotional suppression, and a need to remain composed. No one had really had the space to process much. They functioned and survived, but they carried it, and the body reflected this.

The pelvis and lower spine can often hold themes related to survival, control, stability, trusting others and our environment, and at times unexpressed emotional load. In her case, it felt less like a reaction and more like a long-standing adaptation that makes sense in relation to ancestral trauma.

Through Spinal Energetics, that area gradually softened as her system began to reorganize. Not in a dramatic way, but steadily over time. The holding reduced, her breath dropped lower, and the pressure through her lower back eased.

What changed wasn't just the pain for her, it was that her body no longer needed to maintain the same level of containment.

When a pattern is that stable, that consistent, and that disconnected from current circumstances in the person's life, it often points beyond the individual and the current times. The body has learnt to organize itself over time and sometimes, that organization didn't begin with them.

CHAPTER 9

LIVED EXPERIENCES AND OUTDATED STORIES

While the ancestral software and early-childhood blueprints provide the foundation, the most visceral chapters of our story are written through lived experiences. This is the data we input ourselves—the code generated by our direct trauma (big, little and chronic), the choices we make, the roles we adopt to survive the world, and the moments that taught us who we are (accurate or not).

If our DNA is the software, then our lived experiences are the daily updates and manual entries we type into our system. Every interaction we have is a data point. From the way a barista looks at us in the morning to the tone of a partner's voice, our brain is constantly scanning for information to either confirm or deny the stories we have already told ourselves.

We rarely see the world as it is; we see the world as we are.

If your internal story is, "I am not seen," you will subconsciously overlook the five people who smiled at you and focus entirely on the one person who didn't hold the door open. That single interaction becomes "proof" that your story is true. Your brain hits "Enter" on that line of code, and it becomes more deeply embedded in your biology. Over time, these reinforced stories become our truth, even if they are based on a faulty original premise.

This process is driven by confirmation bias—a psychological phenomenon that acts as the algorithm for our internal search engine. Our brains are bombarded with billions of bits of information every second. To prevent a total system crash, the brain creates filters to prioritize what it deems relevant. If you have coded yourself with the belief that you are unworthy or unsupported, your confirmation bias will aggressively seek out evidence to support that belief while actively discarding evidence to the contrary.

This creates a self-fulfilling prophecy. When we expect to be let down, we often act in ways that protect us from being let down—perhaps by being distant or defensive—which then causes others to pull away. When they pull away, we say, *See? I knew I couldn't lean on anyone.*

This isn't just a mental loop; it is a physical one. Each time the bias is confirmed, the nervous system sends a signal to the body to "armor up." The shoulders rise, the breath shallows, and the spine stiffens. We are literally building a wall of bone and tension to support a story that our mind has decided is absolute truth.

The Evolution of the Narrative: Necessary Versus Outdated

It is vital to understand that many of the stories we carry—even the false ones—did not start as errors. They started as highly intelligent survival strategies. Our innate intelligence is always prioritizing safety over growth. When we experience a traumatic event, the body creates a narrative to ensure that we never have to experience that specific pain again.

Take, for example, a woman who was sexually assaulted by a man. In the immediate aftermath, her survival instinct will write a protective narrative: "All men are a threat. All men are dangerous." This narrative is not wrong; it is a necessary, life-saving overcorrection. Her nervous system is keeping her in a state of hypervigilance to ensure her physical survival, and her body will physically reflect this. She may carry immense tension in her psoas and pelvic floor, her lumbar spine may flatten to brace her foundation, and her energy will likely feel retracted or shielded. This is her innate intelligence doing its job perfectly.

However, as time passes and she moves into a different, safer chapter of her life, that same narrative—which was once her greatest protector—becomes her greatest cage. While her body is reacting in a way that is entirely conducive to her past experiences, it is not a reaction that is helpful for her future growth. When it comes to nurturing relationships with men, the code that says "all men are threats" will prevent her from ever feeling the safety required to build healthy relationships. The story has now become an outdated narrative—a piece of code that was vital for a specific crisis but has now become a chronic glitch in her system.

The Cost of the Outdated Story

We carry thousands of these outdated stories.

- The story that you must be "the funny one" to be liked leaves you with a neck that is constantly strained from wearing a mask.
- The story that "money is hard to find" keeps your lower back in a state of perpetual, unsupported ache.
- The story that "my voice doesn't matter" results in a throat and cervical spine that feel perpetually constricted.

We are often living in a body that is braced for a trauma that ended ten years ago. We are using valuable energetic resources to maintain a protective strategy for a version of ourselves that no longer exists. This is why we feel exhausted, disconnected, and in chronic pain.

It's also why a lot of clients experience the "straw that broke the camel's back" type injuries. I often see clients who are utterly perplexed by their pain. They might say, "Sarah, I was just bending over to pick up a pen and my back seized. I'm fit, I do yoga—how can a pen do this?"

It wasn't the pen. It was the fact that you were already at 99 percent capacity.

We live in a culture that rewards the hustle. We are taught to push through and prioritize productivity over presence. Every time you ignored your body's need for rest, every time you swallowed your anger to keep the peace, and every time you stayed in a situation that felt off, you added another drop of stress to an increasingly overloaded capacity.

The pen was simply the final drop that forced the system into a "protective strategy." When the nervous system decides it can no longer handle the load, it creates a physical outcome—a spasm, a knot, or a locked joint—to stop you from moving further into danger. The pain is not an error in the sense that your body is failing; it is a highly intelligent survival mechanism that is trying to communicate to you that something needs your attention.

National Codes

We also live in national story codes. From your town to your state and your country, the societal attitudes and beliefs held by each will subconsciously dictate your code. Even if our own households hold differing beliefs, we are exposed to broader values through school, the community and media—meaning the values, beliefs and attitudes that our countries are built on are an almost inescapable facet of our development and ongoing lives.

In Australia, our national identity is built on the myth of the "laid-back larrikin." We are the country of thongs, barbecues, and the effortless "she'll be right" attitude. But if you look at the clinical data, a different story emerges. We are a nation carrying some of the highest levels of personal debt on the planet. This creates a fascinating somatic paradox: the "Casual Mask."

We project a relaxed, open upper body to the world, but the lower half of the body—the lumbar spine and the pelvis—tells the truth. It is locked in a state of "survival bracing." Because our homes are often our greatest source of both pride and peril, our foundation (the lower back) is constantly preparing for a fall that hasn't happened yet.

Additionally, our convict heritage has left us with a deep-seated, collective belief in egalitarianism—which sounds noble until it manifests as Tall Poppy Syndrome. In Australia, there is a subconscious pressure to remain "level" with the pack. If you stand too tall, if you are too ambitious, or if you express too much pride in your success, the cultural "clippers" come out to prune you back down to size.

Physically, this acts as a somatic ceiling. I see it in high-achieving clients who, despite their success, carry a subtle hunch or a collapse in their thoracic spine. It is the posture of a person trying not to be noticed. They are literally "toning down" their energetic presence to avoid being ostracized. Their innate intelligence has decided that it is safer to be mediocre and included than to be exceptional and alone.

Every country has its own version of this based on its national values and attitudes.

In the United States, there is the relentless pressure of the "American Dream"—the belief that you can, and should, be anything you want if you just work hard enough. This creates a nation of people leaning perpetually into the future. Physically, this manifests as a forward-head posture and a hyper-reactive nervous system; it is the posture of the hunter, always reaching for the next achievement, the next "more," and never quite landing in the present moment.

In Japan, the cultural emphasis on *Wa* (harmony) and the collective over the individual can lead to a literal suppression of the self. There is a deep-seated stoicism and an extreme work ethic—captured by the term *Karoshi*: death from overworking. In the spine, this often appears as a rounding of the shoulders and a bowing of the upper back (the thoracic heart space), as the individual shrinks their own needs and expressions to fit into the rigid requirements of the group.

In the United Kingdom, the "stiff upper lip" is more than just a phrase; it is a somatic reality. For generations, the British have been taught that emotional outbursts are "bad form" and that one must simply carry on regardless of internal distress. This results in a massive amount of tension held in the jaw (TMJ) and the cervical spine. It is the physical act of swallowing one's truth, leading to a neck that is rigid and a voice that is energetically constricted.

Whether it is the pressurized hustle of New York or the selflessness of Japan, we are all products of our "National Code" and that contributes to the overall story we carry.

Intergenerational Wisdom

On the other hand, it's important to note that the spine doesn't only record our trauma; it also records our triumphs. When we are in alignment—when our soul and our external circumstances are the same—the spine reflects this. We also carry the stories that are wise, strong and resilient.

Think of a time when you felt truly proud, truly "at home" in yourself. Your chest was open, your chin was level, and your spine felt long and effortless. This is when you are in alignment and are balanced. A healthy spine is not one that is perfectly straight (that's just another form of rigidity); it is a spine that can move. It can be strong when it needs to protect, and it can be soft when it needs to connect.

Spinal Energetics looks at your deeper stories, not just the intergenerational trauma but the intergenerational wisdom. We have an intelligent system and it's always trying to keep us aligned and safe. We need to acknowledge that there is something fundamentally right about our bodies' wisdom.

It craves wellness and wholeness. It wants healing and restoration, flexibility and peace. The body does all it can to protect, nourish and care for you.

Lin's Case Study

One of my clients Lin is the perfect illustration of this. Lin came to me with ultra-tight muscles and back tension. He told me that he did his flexibility exercises and watched his stress levels. While talking to me, he said his parents came from China and did "backbreaking" work their whole lives to give him opportunities they never had. It struck me that he used that terminology. I probed deeper. It turns out that Lin felt guilty about the backbreaking work of his parents, and he carried that load on his body. He felt it was his responsibility to carry it.

Over a few sessions we worked on the load Lin was carrying. He began to see the relationship between his parents' sacrifice and his own pain. After reframing his parents' work into something that revealed their strength and resilience, Lin's spine began to shift into alignment. He moved from a painful story to a powerful story simply through the language he used and the lens he looked through.

Leading American psychiatrist and co-author of *What Happened to You?* Dr. Bruce Perry says our relatedness is often the medicine we need. He emphasizes that healing requires safe, attuned, and consistent relationships over time, which are often lacking in the modern, rushed environment. He says, "Connectedness has the power to counterbalance adversity."

I believe connection is key. Connection to ourselves, our stories, our tribes, our communities, our bodies, and our hearts and souls.

CHAPTER 10

THE MODERN DILEMMA

WIRED AND TIRED

This brings us to the final contributing factor to our stories: the current time we live in, meaning the 21st century and more specifically 2026. The context we are operating in is very different from the ones our parents had and different even to those living in other areas of the world. From the societal expectations around a woman's role to the 40-hour work week, definitions of success, and the death of the village, everything that happens around us contributes to the stories we tell ourselves about who we are, and more potently, *who we think we should be*.

Even more than that, the technological advancements of the last 20 years have meant an unprecedented increase in information availability, meaning that there is now a catastrophic amount of input that is overwhelming for an individual to process.

Your spine is the antenna that receives this social context, expectations and stimulus, constantly reading and responding to the frequencies of the world around you. And quite frankly, the frequency of the modern world is overstimulating as fuck. We are not only operating with decades of conflicting history, we are also operating within a current societal context that our biological systems simply weren't designed to handle.

Non-Conducive Work Models

When it comes to the way our society is structured fundamentally in terms of work and economic function, we are still living under the shadow of the Industrial Revolution. The pervasive 40-hour work week did not descend from the heavens as a divine law of human productivity. It was a compromise born of the early 20th century and a product of much harsher working conditions.

Before the mid-1800s, human rhythm was dictated by the sun and the seasons. We worked in bursts and rested in cycles, and our sleep patterns used to be biphasic, meaning people used to go to sleep shortly after dusk for about four hours before waking up and having a two-hour period of wakefulness where they would read, talk or pray. Then they would go back to sleep for another four hours and wake up at dawn. Work was fundamentally task-oriented rather than time-oriented; people worked in intense bursts when the harvest required it and retreated into long periods of rest and repair during the winter months.

However, the rise of factories demanded a linear, predictable output. As the Industrial Revolution reached its peak, men, women and children were frequently subjected to 12-to-16-hour workdays in hazardous, sunless conditions. This era saw a total collapse of the ancestral sleep and movement cycles, forcing the nervous system into a state of chronic exhaustion. After decades of labor movements fighting for "eight hours for work, eight hours for rest, and eight hours for what we will," Henry Ford popularized the 40-hour week for his automotive workers in the 1920s. He didn't do it for their well-being; he did it because he realized that overworked people made mistakes and didn't have enough leisure time to buy the cars they were making.

The 40-hour work week is still the standard for most, and while there are significant moves to reduce this further, the fact remains that right now our bodies are being forced into a pattern that is not natural or beneficial to our physical, mental and emotional health.

The human spine is a masterpiece of mobility. It thrives on movement, variety, and the frequent shifting of weight. Yet, the modern 40-hour week demands the one thing the spine hates most: stasis.

We spend the vast majority of our eight hours of work in chairs. This is not just a postural problem; it is a physiological crisis. When you sit for eight hours, you are essentially asking your body to go into hibernation while your brain is expected to perform at peak capacity. This creates a massive energetic bottleneck. The energy is all in the head while the rest of the body is starved of circulation and movement.

A common narrative is that we can out-train our desk jobs. However, the science of sedentary behavior tells a much darker story. Research has shown that prolonged sitting is an independent risk factor for disease. This means that the damage caused by sitting for eight hours a day cannot be undone by a morning workout. One study published in the *Annals of Internal Medicine* found that even for those who exercise regularly, the negative health effects of prolonged sitting—including metabolic issues and cardiovascular risk—remain significant.

Beyond this lies an even more fundamental misalignment: the model is built entirely around male physiology. The traditional workday assumes a 24-hour hormonal cycle—a rhythm that mirrors the male testosterone peak in the morning and its gradual decline by evening. For a body operating on this 24-hour clock, a linear, repetitive daily structure makes biological sense. However, those with a female biology are also governed by an infradian rhythm—a 28-day (approximate) cycle that affects brain chemistry, metabolism and the immune system.

The modern workplace demands that women be the same person every day at 9:00 a.m., regardless of whether they are in their follicular phase (high energy, expansive) or their luteal phase (retracted, restorative). By ignoring the complexity of the menstrual cycle, women are forced to override their innate intelligence for three out of every four weeks and this creates a surge in cortisol.

This is applicable to everyone though, as human beings are

inherently cyclical, not mechanical. Regardless of gender, our focus and energy levels are governed by ultradian rhythms—biological cycles that repeat throughout the 24-hour day, typically lasting 90 to 120 minutes. At the end of a cycle, the body naturally craves a period of rest and recalibration. However, the 9-to-5 industrial model ignores these peaks and valleys, demanding a flat, consistent output that simply doesn't exist in biology.

When we force ourselves to "push through" these natural dips in energy—often fueled by caffeine or looming deadlines—we are effectively overriding our nervous system. We are signaling to the body that it is not safe to rest. To maintain this unnatural state of alertness, the body recruits the sympathetic nervous system (fight-or-flight), flooding the system with cortisol and adrenaline just to get through a Tuesday afternoon.

Over time, this chronic overriding of our energetic boundaries manifests as physical density. The spine, which should be a flexible conduit for energy, becomes a storage unit for this unspent survival stress. This is the genesis of some idiopathic pain. It is the physical accumulation of all the times we said "go" when our body said "stop."

Ultimately, a work model that demands we act like machines leaves us dangerously susceptible to burnout and emotional injury. Burnout is not just the result of doing "too much"; it is the result of living in a way that is fundamentally at odds with our design. When we sever the connection to our natural rhythms, we lose our resilience, leaving us brittle, exhausted, and disconnected from the very vessel we live in.

Shifting Social Roles

One of the most profound societal shifts throughout the past 100 years has been the change in gender roles. To truly understand where we are now, we must explore a brief history of where we've been.

- **Pre-Industrial Era:** Gender roles were fluid and integrated, with men and women operating as communal co-laborers whose work followed the natural, task-oriented rhythms of the sun and the seasons.
- **Early Industrial Revolution:** The demands of early factory life forced men, women, and children into the same brutal 16-hour workdays.
- **Mid 19th Century:** The British Parliament (and subsequently other Western nations) began passing Factory Acts to protect children, but they quickly expanded to include "protected persons"—namely, women. While these laws were framed as humanitarian, they had a secondary effect: they restricted the hours women could work and the types of jobs they could hold. This made women less "hirable" than men. In the eyes of the law, women were being recategorized from productive workers to vulnerable dependents.
- **Victorian/Late Industrial Era:** Male-dominated labor unions began to push for what they called a "Family Wage." Their argument was that a man should be paid enough to support a wife and children at home. This saw the deliberate creation of the "Male Breadwinner" and

the "Angel in the House," where the male became the sole provider while the woman was recategorized as the domestic caregiver. If a man's wife had to work, it was seen as a sign of his failure as a provider. While the working class was dealing with wages, the Victorian middle class was creating the values code known as the Cult of Domesticity.

- **The 1950s:** While the two World Wars briefly forced women back into the factories, the post-WWII era saw a desperate attempt to return to "normalcy." The 1950s took the Victorian ideal and supercharged it with consumerism. The Nuclear Family became a tool of the Cold War—a symbol of Western stability. This is when the "Stay-at-Home Mom" became a suburban requirement.
- **The Late 20th Century (1960s–1990s):** Second-wave feminism brought the mass entry of women into higher education and professional careers, a transition that challenged the domestic role, but simultaneously birthed the "Double Burden," as women began to navigate the workforce without a corresponding shift in societal or household support.
- **The Modern Era (2026):** Men and women have equal representation in the workforce, yet the balance is not quite perfect in terms of household management and child rearing. Even in progressive homes, research shows that women still take on the majority of the domestic labor, the emotional labor of managing relationships, and the

> logistical labor of raising children. This is made worse by societal infrastructure failures, such as parental leave being primarily offered to women only (meaning they have no choice but to be the primary caregiver lest they forfeit their family's leave entitlements). This means that even though the roles look equal from far away, a closer look sees a strain on women to "have it all" and does not give men much choice in their role of the breadwinner.

From a Spinal Energetics perspective, both men and women suffer from the aftereffects of the societal pressures and changing roles that have occurred in the past decades. A lot of men have this strong desire to be the breadwinner and provide for their families even though they've grown up in a time where women were studying and working alongside them. This could be passed down in the "code" from their great-grandfather—who was required to be the sole provider. Women on the other hand, have had the most radical changes, swinging from one side of the pendulum to the other. It's no wonder women have grown up either believing that they have to "do it all" or they have to choose between a family and career. There's been periods of time where each reality has existed, and our bodies don't forget that very easily.

Therefore, not only are we dealing with the *current* societal values and beliefs about the roles of men and women, but we also have decades of change imprinted in our inherited codes that often creates friction and misalignment. This can make it harder to push past the "noise" and tap into what our soul truly wants and craves.

The Death of the Village

We were designed to live in multi-generational communities, embedded in a "village" that shared the load of child-rearing and had elders who offered wisdom and a stabilizing presence. However, today—particularly in the Western world—we live in nuclear silos. We have traded the village for privacy and independence, and the cost is a massive increase in individual pressure.

When the village disappears, the lumbar spine—the energetic seat of support—begins to fail.

To understand why this happens, we have to look at the nuance of what we are missing. In the 1970s, sociologist Robert S. Weiss developed the "Relational Theory of Loneliness," which offers a profound insight into our modern condition.[54] Weiss argued that loneliness isn't a singular experience; rather, there are two distinct types of provisions we need to feel whole: emotional integration and social integration.

Emotional integration usually comes from our intimate attachments—a partner, a spouse, or a parent. Social integration, however, comes from a network of shared concerns—a community, a tribe, or a village. Weiss discovered that you cannot simply swap one for the other. You can be happily married (emotionally integrated) and still feel a desperate, gnawing sense of isolation if you lack a community (socially isolated).

This is the crisis of the modern family. We have placed the entire weight of the village onto the shoulders of our partners and our immediate households. We are trying to get our needs for social integration met by a single person, and when that inevitably fails, we feel unsupported.

This isolation is compounded by the "Stranger Danger" culture that emerged in the late 20th century. We taught children to fear anyone they didn't know, which inadvertently broke the back of spontaneous community interaction. It is rare now that we chat with our neighbor or the person next to us at the park. We are hyper-connected via our smartphones yet profoundly disconnected in our physical reality.

The contrast is stark when we look at some of the "Blue Zones"—regions of the world where people live the longest and healthiest lives. In these cultures, people are not segregated from society but they have developed close-knit communities where everyone has a place of belonging. They have an authentic role to play, and they help one another in times of need. In the Blue Zone of Sardinia, Italy, for example, there is a tradition where the community pools their money together. If someone falls ill or faces hardship, the village resources take care of them. There is a direct, tangible level of support and love that simply doesn't happen on a large scale in our individualized societies.

Sure, we may have welfare systems (and these are extremely important), but they are often impersonal or resented by those who do not see the value in it. And even if we do have family and friends to lean on, there is a stigma attached to needing help.

In modern society, we are toxically independent and expected to always be fully self-sufficient. If you are supported, you are viewed as "spoiled" or weak.

As a result, we are missing the safety net—the social integration—that directly affects our internal ability to feel safe, secure, and like we belong, and that's why we are seeing both a rise in loneliness and burnout. I don't believe these are two separate things. The burnout is coming from our loneliness and the exhaustion of trying to be a village of just one or two.

Societal Constructs

In Western cultures—Australia, the UK, the US—our definition of success has become increasingly externalized. We are raised on a diet of "more": more money, more property, more accolades, more options. We are taught that the path to happiness is a checklist: go to university, get the high-paying job, buy the house, get the golden retriever, and secure the perfect partner.

Yet, in my practice, I see a recurring and troubling pattern. People walk through my door who have ticked every single box. They have done everything they were told would make them happy and they have security, status and material comfort. And yet, they are profoundly empty.

They are confused because the formula didn't work. They are suffering from a misalignment—a widening gap between who they are on a soul level and who they have become to survive in society.

Part of this modern malaise stems from what psychologist Barry Schwartz coined "The Paradox of Choice."[55] We assume that more freedom means more happiness, but infinite choice often leads to paralysis and dissatisfaction.

Think of it like a restaurant menu. If you go to a place with five excellent dishes, you choose the chicken, and you enjoy it. But if you go to a restaurant with a ten-page menu offering 200 options, the experience changes. You choose the chicken, but you spend the entire meal wondering if you should have had the steak, or the pasta, or the fish. The sheer volume of possibility breeds anxiety and the fear of missing out.

We see this everywhere now—from the 70 shades of nail polish at the salon to the endless swipe-right nature of modern dating. In previous generations, options were limited. My mother, for example, had far fewer career paths available to her than I do. This isn't to say that limitation is better or that we should romanticize the past's lack of opportunity for women, but there was a certain psychological safety in simplicity. When the goalposts aren't constantly moving, it is easier to find contentment.

Today, we are drowning in opportunity, which of course is an extremely privileged position to have, but it has created a new kind of pressure: the pressure to be everything, all at once. We're told to go to university and get a well-paying job, but then you're also expected to have traveled extensively and lived abroad and bought a house and a car and a dog, but also that you should invest in your creativity and get a job that is *fulfilling* and not worry about money, and yet if you're not making enough money, why don't you just choose a different career? There are so many different versions of ourselves available that it can feel like a failure no matter what you choose because you're denying the other five options.

On top of this, there are the micro-expectations to be the perfect parent, the perfect partner, the perfect employee and the perfect version of ourselves at all times.

The result is a society that is wired but tired. We are stuck in a state of high-functioning anxiety, constantly adding to our to-do lists in a desperate attempt to optimize our lives, while drifting further and further away from our internal compass.

This internal friction often manifests specifically in the cervical spine (the neck). There's usually tension in the upper neck and it's a pattern or painful spot on one side that is recurring. A lot of people come in and say, "Oh yeah, my chiropractor always has to adjust that same spot over and over and over again."

It's always that spot, and if we are returning to the same environment that created it in the first place, then it's always going to come back. The body's communicating to you that what you're doing is not true success for you, whether that's because you are living your life for someone else, in a way that is for pure advancement or materialism, or striving for perfectionism out of a fear of failure. I refer to this as the mental aspect of the ego—often called the "monkey mind." It is that restless, chattering voice that constantly swings from one thought to the next, analyzing and over-complicating everything. For many people, this monkey mind is the only pilot flying the plane. It creates so much mental static that they lose touch with their true self, to the point where they don't even know what they genuinely like anymore—only what the noise tells them they should like.

These are the clients who cannot switch off. They need the TV on to relax; they need background noise to study. They are terrified of silence because silence invites the truth, and that truth might be inconvenient.

The truth might be that they hate being a doctor even though they spent ten years studying for it, or that their marriage looks perfect on Instagram but feels lonely in real life, or that the friendship group they've had for 20 years drains them.

This is the battle between the soul and the social expectations. The spine becomes rigid because the person is holding themselves together, bracing against the reality of their own unhappiness.

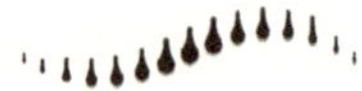

When we look to the East, there is a lot of diversity in the societal ideals of success. The energetic signature of a salaryman in Tokyo is vastly different from that of a rice farmer in Bali or a monk in Thailand. However, despite these regional nuances, the East generally operates under a collectivist framework, whereas the West operates under an individualist one.

In countries like Japan or South Korea, there is immense societal pressure to have successful careers, but it is often rooted in family honor and duty rather than the Western pursuit of individual glory or material accumulation. The stress there is real, but it has a different flavor—it is the stress of obligation rather than the stress of ambition.

In contrast, when I travel to Buddhist communities in Southeast Asia or parts of India, I see an energetic signature that is profoundly different from what we see in my clinic back in Australia. Their survival needs are often pressing—many are living day to day—and their drive is rarely materialistic. Their success is internal. It is based on community, contribution, and energetic integrity.

This difference in mindset creates a different manifestation in the body. In the West, we see a prevalence of upper cervical tension, but in developing Eastern communities, the tension often sits lower. We see issues in the lumbar spine (the root chakra), which correlates to survival, safety, and financial stability. We also see physical deformities caused by manual labor, malnutrition, or carrying heavy loads. However, despite these physical hardships, there is often less psycho-emotional friction in their spines.

In Spinal Energetics, we operate on a core principle: **The greater the distance between your reality and your soul, the greater the tension in your spine.**

In the West, we are in a constant state of resistance. We think life *should* be different than it is. We believe we should be richer, thinner, or happier and our soul needs are often the sacrifice in pursuit of these things. This resistance creates a chaotic frequency in the nervous system—a dissonance between the soul and the ego.

In many Eastern cultures, particularly those influenced by Buddhist or Hindu philosophies, there is a higher level of acceptance. There is a surrender to what is, and because there is less mental resistance to their reality, the energy flows more freely. They may have physical pain from hard work, but they often lack the rigid, armored quality that comes from suppressing the soul's truth.

This lack of resistance extends to how emotions are processed collectively.

When I went to the Philippines though it was a little bit different. I did volunteer work in primary schools and the issues were more emotional because a lot of them had lost parents or family members. However, what was interesting is that it wasn't showing up so much in their spine as a discourse—it was just another layer to move through. And what was beautiful is they all held each other's hands if one cried and there was no embarrassment around emotional vulnerability or display. So again, no friction. It was able to just flow. Whereas here in the West, if a child was crying, it would be quite rare to see other kids hold their hand and cry with them at the sadness of that feeling.

It was a profound display of communal regulation, and because the emotion was allowed to be expressed, validated, and shared, it didn't need to be stored.

When you suppress an emotion to maintain social acceptability, that energy does not disappear. The law of conservation of energy states that energy cannot be created or destroyed, only transformed. So, when you swallow your grief or your anger, it transforms into tension. It settles into the fascia, the muscles, and the vertebrae. It waits.

Bronnie Ware, an Australian palliative care nurse who spent years with patients in their final weeks, recorded their most common regrets in her book *The Top Five Regrets of the Dying*. The top two were:

1. "I wish I'd had the courage to live a life true to myself, not the life others expected of me."
2. "I wish I hadn't worked so hard."[56]

These regrets are a warning from the future. They are a reminder that the Australian Dream or the American Dream of the white picket fence and the high-stress career is often a trap.

Spinal Energetics is about breaking that trap. It is about clearing the noise of society so you can finally hear your own voice. It is about creating a pause in the endless scroll of choices so you can ask the only question that matters: *Does this path actually belong to me?*

The Global Burden

Perhaps the most damaging part of our modern environment is the death of "local" living. In our ancestors' time, news was what happened in the immediate surroundings. If a house burned down three towns over, they wouldn't hear about it for a month. Their nervous systems were only required to process the stress of their immediate vicinity.

Today, we carry the world's trauma in our pockets.

We wake up and scroll through international news before we've even brushed our teeth. We take on the weight of wars thousands of kilometers away, famines in distant continents, and political upheavals in foreign lands. Our boundaries of consciousness have been expanded to an impossible level.

When you see a graphic image of a conflict on your screen, your HPA axis (the stress response) still fires even though you are safe in your physical surroundings. When something major happens, we are put into a state of secondhand mourning and anxiety that no other generation has experienced. This is not normal. We are trying to process the sorrow of the world with a nervous system designed to process the sorrow of the tribe. Additionally, we have constant access to news, which means our nervous systems rarely get a break. Instead of hearing about global news on the radio at certain times of the day or reading the newspaper, we get notifications at all times of the day and night with detailed information and graphic images and videos.

This expanded consciousness is a distracted consciousness. It decreases our capacity to function in our actually very small, very real lives. It fills our "cup" to 90 percent capacity with things we cannot change, leaving us with decreased resilience for the things we can change. This is why we feel so overwhelmed. Our spines are carrying the weight of the entire world, and it is a weight we were never meant to bear.

CHAPTER 11

The Spine as a Map to Healing and Potential

From the genetic software of your ancestors to the mirrored blueprints of your early childhood, the manual entries of your lived trauma, and the noise of the modern context, there is a massive influx of information that determines who we are.

What all of this means is that the person you are is not just a biological coincidence. You are a living synthesis of a century of stories. Your current physical state—your posture, your persistent aches, your energy levels—is the cumulative "printout" of every layer of code we have discussed. You are carrying a heavy, complex, and often conflicting narrative that has been written into your bones by people you never met, environments you didn't choose, and experiences you were never taught to integrate.

In other words, people are often paying a massive "interest rate" on an energetic debt they didn't accrue.

Imagine your body has a limited amount of currency—the energy required for healing, for creativity, for joy, and for simply living your life. When your system is running outdated software (like an ancestral survival brace or an old protective strategy from a childhood trauma), it is using a huge portion of that currency to maintain those states. You are effectively using 90 percent of your battery to run background apps that you don't even need anymore. This is why you feel exhausted, even when you've slept well, eaten well, exercised and done everything else possible to look after your physical body. The cause of your tiredness, pain, or feeling of "stuckness" might not be physical, it might be coming from one of these many other sources.

The Truth About Idiopathic Pain

This brings us to the heart of why so many people suffer from idiopathic pain—pain that has no clear medical cause or physical explanation.

In the traditional Western model, if an X-ray doesn't show a fracture and a blood test doesn't show inflammation, the pain is often dismissed or managed with band-aid solutions. But in Spinal Energetics, we know that idiopathic pain is rarely a mystery; it is simply a message written in a language most people haven't learned to read.

Your pain is the print error that occurs when the story in your code no longer matches the reality of your soul. For example, that "unexplained" lower back pain is often a lack of support in other areas of your life.

You can't fix idiopathic pain by only looking at the physical matter, because the body is only reacting to the signal. To heal the pain, you have to address the signal—which means you have to address the story.

This is the *why* behind Spinal Energetics. We don't just manipulate bone or massage tissue; we co-facilitate the integration of your history. We work with the spine as the "antenna" because it is the most direct pathway to the innate intelligence—the master engineer of your code.

True healing is about becoming the conscious author of your own code. It's about looking at the stories you've been carrying and deciding which ones are worth keeping and which ones are ready to be integrated and released.

The work of Spinal Energetics is to help the body find true alignment with the soul.

We aren't trying to delete experiences or dismiss "outdated" survival mechanisms; we are trying to understand what the innate intelligence is communicating with us and make changes to put it at ease.

When we work with the spine, we are talking directly to the nervous system. We are saying, *I see why you built this wall. I see how it kept you safe. But you are safe now. You can afford to soften.* By bringing awareness to how our daily interactions and our confirmation biases are keeping these stories alive, we begin to create a gap. In that gap, we can choose a new narrative. The new story is:

"I can move from a state of protection to a state of connection."

You can finally put down the weight of the stories that were never yours to carry.

You can release the stories that are no longer true.

You can say goodbye to the old identities you have outgrown or no longer serve you.

Recognizing these patterns and stories is not about blaming our parents or feeling shame or guilt for past experiences. Nor is it to feel like a victim to circumstances. It is about *context*.

When you realize that your anxiety might be an ancestral survival gift that has simply outlived its usefulness, the shame begins to dissolve. When you understand your tendency to shut down and suppress your feelings as a result of growing up in a household that required this to survive, you realize that these traits are not fixed and just as you learnt these, you can learn others. You realize you aren't "broken" or stuck this way forever; you are simply a highly sophisticated biological super-system running "'software" that no longer matches you on a soul level.

But to get new software, we have to understand the one we're currently working with, which is where Spinal Energetics comes into play.

Listening to Your Higher Self

If I'd shared what I was planning to do with Spinal Energetics, many would have thought it was a dumb idea. I didn't have a big plan, I just wanted to help my clients and I felt an energetic force pulling me toward it.

Before Spinal Energetics, I didn't have a deep soul connection to my work, so I knew what lackluster impulse felt like and how it often resulted in disengagement, burnout, and fatigue. When I started Spinal Energetics, there was less friction and for the first time I experienced what it was like to work hard and *not* get tired. To feel ignited by purpose-led work without burnout.

Over time, I listened to this inner impulse and developed a listening relationship with it. I now know how to deeply listen to my **higher self** and can sense if I'm in a flow or not. When I'm not, I make a change. Success for me is listening to my soul and following through with what it's asking for. As soon as I feel that friction, I know I must pivot.

At one point during my career, traveling the globe with my work was the goal and I loved it. But as soon as I felt that I wasn't loving it as much, I implemented changes to align with my needs (which is a privilege since I own my own business).

Having that relationship with yourself and listening to what your soul is telling you is a powerful tool. Because otherwise there's tension between who you are and your reality. Sometimes the more resistance you feel toward something, the more important that aspect of your life is for your soul. Additionally, it's important to point out that not all tension is "bad." We can use it to push and pull toward the end results that we want and use it almost like a bridge to step from our current reality to the next.

Clients often tell me they live with this tension, and it pushes and pulls them daily. They tell me that they can sense that they are not in flow, or not moving in the right direction or environment but are too scared to make the change. They worry about the outcome of making changes, the potential loss of income, the change of relationships, or identity. The fear of failure. The fear of the unknown.

Their inner knowing may be tapping on their soul but listening to it takes courage. Some people decide to settle, and stagnancy and even sadness seeps in. This creates friction between what the soul wants and your circumstances.

Do you know that feeling? That tug of war between the head and the heart? The friction between your soul's voice and your circumstances? Can you identify what the deeper part of you is calling out?

Most people don't and that's because they're not fully connected to their body or true self. So, when they first come into the clinic, that's where we begin: connection to self. Society's lifestyle and loud narratives often disconnect people from their true soul voice. Society's stories often encourage listening to a fearful or anxious voice. Or a pure analytical and practical voice. The voice we may have been told to listen to in childhood may not even be ours, it could be the voice of our parents telling us what voice "should" be listened to.

The reality is that we have a "committee" of voices in our heads and not every thought passing through your mind comes from your true self, but rather just a temporary event in a complex internal ecosystem. You likely have an anxious voice that frantically drafts worst-case scenarios to keep you safe, or perhaps a critical voice that echoes old pressures and expectations. These thoughts are often automatic reflexes rather than deep truths. It's beneath this chatter that lies the presence of what is often called the "soul voice" or the True Self. This part of you does not judge or panic; it simply watches the thoughts drift by like clouds and only speaks truths straight from the soul or inner intelligence.

While our other voices can be persistent, they are usually fleeting, frantic and driven by fear or insecurities. In contrast, the true soul voice tends to not go away over time and appears when you're in a quiet state with a strong, calm tone. The skill comes in learning to discern between all your different voices, and it can be a profound relief to realize that not every thought is equal or true.

For example, people with OCD often have pervasive and inappropriate intrusive thoughts that can be quite distressing, as they are often directly in conflict with their values. But part of learning to live with OCD is learning what is their anxious "OCD" brain talking and what is their true voice. This is done through cognitive behavioral therapy, rerouting of thought patterns, and something as simple as dismissing the thoughts with a, "That's just my OCD talking, it's not real." Everyone can learn this same kind of discernment and the best way to do this is to get closer to your true self.

Meditation and yoga are two great ways to do this, which were both the two biggest influences on how I learned this. It's just about giving space and time to get to know yourself. As Lao Tzu said, "At the center of your being you have the answer; you know who you are and you know what you want."

I think people fear that inner space. We saw that during the pandemic era when people were forced to stay at home and sit with themselves. That was a very challenging time because people had to ask themselves questions or hear things they may not have wanted to hear.

Here's a clear way you can distinguish between your **Higher Self (True/Soul voice)** and other internal voices:

Differentiating Inner Voices

ASPECT	HIGHER SELF/ SOUL VOICE	FEARFUL/ ANXIOUS VOICE	CRITICAL/ CONDITIONED VOICE
CORE ENERGY	Calm, grounded, steady	Urgent, restless, tense	Tight, harsh, pressuring
TONE	Gentle but clear	Fast, loud, repetitive	Sharp, judgmental
EMOTIONAL QUALITY	Peaceful, reassuring	Fearful, worried	Shame-based, critical
PACE	Slow, spacious	Rapid, spiraling	Repetitive loops
FOCUS	Truth, alignment, growth	Worst-case scenarios, danger	Perfection, expectations, "shoulds"
BODY SENSATION	Relaxation, openness, settled breath	Tight chest, racing heart, unease	Contraction, heaviness, tension
TIMING	Arises in stillness, quiet moments	Triggers under stress or uncertainty	Triggered by comparison, failure, pressure
PERSISTENCE	Consistent over time, doesn't force	Comes in waves, fluctuates	Repeats familiar old patterns
MESSAGE STYLE	Simple, direct, compassionate	Catastrophic, overcomplicated	Harsh, absolute ("you always...," "you never...")
RELATIONSHIP TO YOU	Observes without judgment	Tries to protect you from harm	Tries to control or correct you
TRUTH QUALITY	Feels deeply true and aligned	Feels convincing but unstable	Feels familiar but limiting
AFTER EFFECT	Clarity, relief, grounded action = Expansion	Exhaustion, confusion (Spiral loops and tiredness)	Shame, self-doubt (Stuck in patterns, feels defeated)

Not Every Voice Is Your Soul

Remember, not every voice in your head is *your soul*. You have a whole internal ecosystem—a committee of voices—each trying to serve a purpose. The work isn't to silence them, but to **recognize who's speaking.**

You can ask:

- *Does it feel calm or urgent?*
- *Does it expand me or contract me?*
- *Is it compassionate or critical?*
- *Would this voice speak to someone I love this way?*

If it's calm, clear, and steady → likely **Higher Self.**

If it's loud, fast, or fear-based → likely **protective/ conditioned voice.**

When people "can't hear their Higher Self," it's not because it isn't there, it's because:

- Their nervous system is dysregulated
- Their body isn't yet a safe place to listen from
- Their louder protective voices are dominating

So the first step is **not forcing insight**, but **restoring connection to the body**, where discernment naturally begins.

Discernment in the body means feeling into those physical sensations and your inner somatic wisdom. It's about acknowledging and recognizing somatic signals—such as unease, tummy tightening or tension in the body. The body acts as a physical and spiritual barometer to detect truth, safety, and your Higher Self.

Long-Term Vision and Turning Up the Volume

Knowing whether a voice is aligned with the bigger picture is really important. Short-term doubt or confusion is often part of the process of gaining clarity, but keeping your vision set on the long-term is important so you don't give up on your true destiny.

When I was studying chiropractic at university, there were many moments when I wanted to quit. I didn't enjoy it and it didn't feel aligned at the time. And sometimes, it genuinely wasn't. But when I zoomed out, I knew it *was* aligned with the bigger picture of where I was going. The future me.

So I chose to stay, even though there was friction for those five years. I only pushed through because I could feel that deeper, soul-based alignment underneath it all. And as soon as I graduated and could finally do the work I wanted to do, it was a huge relief. I remember thinking, *thank God I didn't quit.*

We need to be sure we don't mistake the uncomfortable or negative thoughts for a full-body "this isn't right for me" experience. Discernments and context matter.

It's the same in relationships. There can be moments where your protective voice says, "This isn't the person for me" or "I don't want this anymore." But that may reflect how you feel in that moment, not the deeper truth.

The soul voice sounds different. It's clearer, steadier, and not reactive. When it says, "This isn't for me anymore," it comes from a deeper place of knowing. Having that deeper body awareness is like having an inner compass that is always working for you, directing you toward your highest destiny.

Spinal Energetics is designed to help people reconnect to that inner compass.

In Spinal Energetics, we dial up the volume on what your inner intelligence is communicating—and sometimes that's uncomfortable or confronting.

Even if someone doesn't fully know what to expect in their first session, or feels disconnected from themselves, there's bravery in booking and showing up. Something inside of them senses there's value in it. At the same time, people often feel hesitant. There's an unconscious knowing that something deeper may be uncovered—that they may have to face parts of themselves they've avoided. That can bring up anxiety or uncertainty.

Another important piece is that Spinal Energetics isn't designed to feel relaxing or blissful in the way people might expect from healing. We're often taught that if something is good for us, it should feel good during and after. But that's not always how healing works.

For some people, symptoms or pain can feel stronger after a session. It might seem like things have gotten worse, but what's really happened is an increase in awareness. You're feeling more because you're finally connected. Your current of voltage is working better, and you feel it more.

If you've been disconnected from your body for a long time, that reconnection can feel overwhelming at first. But growth isn't only light and easy. There can be moments of relief and clarity, but also moments that feel messy or heavy. It's important to *not* bypass the hard parts.

Recently, someone who had lost a loved one came to a support group and said they wanted to "heal" their grief. But grief isn't something you immediately fix or heal. It's something you relate to over time. What we *can* do is support the person through that process—creating safety so the body can move through its layers in its own time and in a healthy way. That may lead to more acceptance or peace. But the goal isn't to rush someone to a place where they no longer feel it. It's to help them stay present with their experience in a way that's supportive and integrated.

To overcome an obstacle and get to the other side, it may involve elements of bliss, but also elements of pain. As the saying goes, "No mud, no lotus."

Numbing or bypassing is *not* a way through, but a pretend shortcut around. Working with the murky layers underneath it all births the beauty and majesty of the lotus.

The Greater Good Is the Soul Story

The soul doesn't just choose what's good for you or what will make you happy, it picks your greater good. It knows what will develop you. A lot of humanity's most admirable human beings have been through a lot of pain and challenges. Eddie Jaku, a survivor of several German concentration camps during World War II, had to be in one of the worst situations a person could endure to become the "happiest man on earth." And there's a caveat. It's not that he's happy all the time, it's that he learned and understood the value of life and that created a sense of happiness. He tapped into meaning—*true* meaning: "Happiness does not fall out of the sky; it is in your hands."

The ancient Chinese proverb "Story of the Farmer" tells of a farmer's son whose horse runs away. His neighbors say what bad luck that is. The farmer replies, "Maybe." The next day, the horse returns with more horses and the neighbors exclaim what good fortune it is, and the farmer replies, "Maybe." The farmer's son then falls off a horse and breaks his leg. The neighbors exclaim, "Oh, that's really bad about your son."

The farmer shrugs and once again says, "Maybe."

A week later, every healthy young man is sent to war, except the farmer's son who is exempt because of his broken leg.

The truth is that life is full of complex circumstances and deeming them as "good" or "bad" is not wise. What appears bad may in fact hold the seed of goodness and manifest into something good.

Holding Pain and Purpose in Both Hands

I've experienced this on a major scale with my mum's brain damage. It's been a complex grief for me and horrible in countless ways, but it has also birthed good things.

When my mum was 68, she woke up one day with a slight headache and back pain. She'd never had a major health issue in her life, but she suffered from migraines when she was younger. She assumed it was a migraine and went to sleep early that night. I called her the next day but she didn't answer.

We later found out she was in a hospital around the corner. She had called an ambulance and was unconscious by the time they arrived so they couldn't call anyone to let them know where she was. She ended up in a coma for three months with a rare brain disease called acute demyelinating encephalomyelitis. She was in ICU for a very long time and had to learn how to walk, talk, eat and go to the toilet herself all again.

She has done all those things, but because of the damage in the brain, she's only got about a three- or four-year-old's mentality and a damaged short-term memory, but she has long-term memory. So she remembers who I am, which is beautiful, but the main issues are in her frontal lobe, which is also very interesting because the frontal lobe is where a lot of our conditioning happens.

My mum never hugged me growing up; she'd say she loved me every now and then, but not much. She wasn't that kind of woman. She's Dutch and was raised in the stereotypical stoicism of not showing emotion. But now, she runs to give me a hug and says, "I love you. I love you." The conditioning of what she was taught in life is no longer there. She expresses love like an innocent child. It's beautiful.

In children, there's no barrier between who they are and what they express. As we get older, that barrier becomes larger, and we develop filters for socially acceptable behavior. We develop skills to try and read what people are feeling and thinking because we don't show emotions the same. We become socialized to garner an appropriate response or even manipulate body language. If a kid doesn't get a treat, they have a tantrum on the floor, but as adults, when we don't get something that we want in life, we're taught to hold our feelings in. While sociable behavior is obviously a good thing in many aspects, it can be a disservice when it's not authentic and we suppress our emotions to be palatable, accepted, or "mature."

Suppression of authentic feelings manifests in the spine as well.

My mum has been in aged care for years now, and it's been a complex grief. I never considered the type of grief that happens when you lose the person you knew and loved while they are still alive. I was 32 when it happened and essentially it left me feeling like an orphan.

When I speak to my mum, I speak to her soul essence because I don't feel like the mum I knew and was raised by is really there. She doesn't look or sound like the mum I knew. My mum is alive but not fully there. The grief is complicated. It's hovering in a strange limbo where you can't fully grieve the loss of the person and yet you do.

It's also taught me many beautiful things. I have a greater appreciation for life and the fragility of it—it's given me an urgency and a passion for living. I am grateful for my health every single day and that helps me show up as a better person in my life and work.

Some people assume that given the work I do I must be fully healed, and while I do prioritize healing and my relationship with Self, it's not always easy. Life's always going to change and alter, and there's always new things to work through. But I'm good at knowing when I'm disconnected and prioritizing connection.

As I evolve as a person, I also evolve as a practitioner and help others who have complex issues. It's like a resonance occurs in the field—the client and their body or soul can sense that I have some understanding of them on that deeper level.

It's like if you're speaking with a psychologist who hasn't experienced what you're going through. They can hear what you're saying and have a mental understanding of what you're experiencing, but there's a disconnect and lack of soul knowing.

I think having these experiences creates an unspoken safety—it creates a resonance of being in a safe and non-judgmental environment. There's nothing quite as healing as spending time with someone who has felt pain like you. It's the concept of the wounded healer coined by psychiatrist Carl Jung. He described a helper (therapist, doctor, or mentor) who uses their own past wounds or challenges to help others heal.

People try their whole life to be perfect at everything and do everything right, but the most disconnected you can be is to appear as being perfect. Humans don't like perfection. We like imperfection, yet we spend our whole life fighting it.

But here's the thing. Your true self isn't chasing perfection or the illusion of it. Only your ego is. For example, I was once on a 20-hour flight and the TV was down. I had a mini meltdown because it was a long-haul flight before I put it in perspective. I was flying in the air, so with or without a TV, it was a huge privilege in the first place and a very luxurious "problem" to have.

We're so used to convenience and getting our expectations met that we have forgotten it's not our soul that's unhappy; it's the other part of us. So being able to recognize when we're not in our soul becomes more critical than before.

Like if someone cuts me off in traffic and I get angry and swear, I try to quickly realize, okay, that's not me. My humanness is being triggered and that's normal but the deepest part of me is untouched and unharmed. Self-compassion is important; perfection is not.

I found that hard at first as a practitioner. I felt I had to show up perfectly for my clients and say all the right things. It was a lot of pressure, but it wasn't from my soul though. It was from the human side of me that made up a story about other people's expectations.

Both aspects operate inside of us, after all, we are both *human* and *beings.* Our species' name even reflects it. Therefore, it's natural to feel this tug inside of us, and neither are wrong. They are holding the same beautiful person—which is you. But in society, we have leaned heavily on our human aspect and often neglected the being aspect. We must pay homage to the fact they dance gloriously inside of us together.

Having a strong distinction between thoughts and stories spinning around in your head versus the deep inner knowing of your soul can bring a level of peace and clarity. There's a lot of bravery in getting to know yourself at a deeper level and in recognizing the whole nature you have and are.

Spinal Energetics makes the connection of your inner antennae louder, which makes it easier to distinguish if it's your Higher Self or your monkey mind. This becomes your North Star; your compass to help you navigate between truth and falsehood, outer demands and inner needs and your true destiny versus society's expectations. It helps you listen to your wisdom rather than someone else's.

The noise of the world speaks loudly, whereas the voice of the soul whispers softly inside you.

CHAPTER 12

Listening to Your Spine

The Pillars of Somatic Reconnection

Healing is not something we force; it's the innate nature we work with. It begins the moment you stop trying to fix your body's problems and start listening to them. As we've explored, your body is not working against you—it's communicating with you. Every sensation, every area of tension, every shift in posture is part of a language that has been quietly speaking your entire life.

The question is not: *how do I get rid of this?* But, *what is this trying to show me? What have I been holding that's not authentically me?*

As we explored earlier, the spine holds your story. It reflects where you have held on, where you have protected yourself, and where you have adapted to survive. Healing isn't intended to erase your stories but to honor and update your relationship to them. It is the translator of your inner and outer journey and the conduit toward alignment with your mind, body and spirit.

Spinal Energetics practitioners feel and listen to the layers of energy in a somatic way. Our practitioners are facilitators of *your* healing, but they are not the healer. You can begin to heal yourself through restoring your connection to yourself, your body, and your spiritual awareness. Reconnection restores energy and keeps the body in natural flow and movement. The body will heal itself if given the right environment to thrive and renew.

Reconnection

As the central point to our physical system, the spine is the structural communication highway between the brain and body and is closely linked with the fascia network. It also acts as the bridge between the conscious and unconscious mind; in other words, it is the ultimate highway to healing.

The nervous system is constantly scanning for safety or threat, so every experience you've had—especially unresolved or overwhelming ones—gets encoded not just mentally, but physically. When the system perceives something that it can't fully process, it adapts by creating protective responses. These responses become tension patterns in the body.

That's where fascia comes in. Fascia is the connective tissue that wraps around muscles, organs, and the spine—it's continuous throughout the entire body. It doesn't just provide structure; it also stores and transmits information, including stress, emotion, and movement patterns. Because fascia is richly connected to the nervous system, it becomes a kind of physical map of your history.

Over time, repeated protective responses from the nervous system become habitual tension patterns in the fascia. These might show up as:

- Tightness or restriction in certain areas
- Limited movement or fluidity
- Holding patterns that feel "normal" but are compensations

When a practitioner works with the spine, they're interacting with the nervous system in a way that invites awareness and safety. As the nervous system begins to feel safe enough, it can start to:

- Shift out of protective states
- Allow stored tension in the fascia to unwind
- Reorganize patterns that are no longer needed

This is why you might see spontaneous movements, waves, or releases during a session. These aren't random—they're the body's way of discharging stored energy and reorganizing itself. So the reconnection looks like this:

THE NERVOUS SYSTEM CREATES
PROTECTIVE RESPONSES.

THOSE RESPONSES BECOME
STORED AS TENSION PATTERNS.

THE FASCIA HOLDS AND DISTRIBUTES THOSE
PATTERNS THROUGHOUT THE BODY.

SPINAL ENERGETICS WORKS THROUGH THE
SPINE AND FIELD TO HELP THE SYSTEM
RECOGNIZE, RELEASE, AND REORGANIZE.

You can see examples of those shifts here:

Rewired for Life

The spinal shift isn't about fixing the body over and over. It's about helping the system recognize that it no longer needs to stay in those protective loops.

You can think of it like this: The brain and spine are constantly updating based on what they perceive to be true. If your system has learned that the world (or your internal experience) isn't fully safe, it will prioritize protection—tension, guarding, bracing, overthinking. That becomes the "default code." Rewiring happens when the system starts to experience something different, such as safety, awareness, and the ability to process what was previously held.

This is how that shift begins:

1. **Awareness changes the pattern**
   When you bring conscious awareness to your body—noticing tension, breath, subtle movement—you're interrupting automatic loops. The brain starts to receive new information: *this pattern is being seen now, it's not unconscious anymore.*
2. **Safety allows release**
   The nervous system won't let go of tension just because you want it to. It lets go when it feels safe enough. Practices that regulate the system—slow breath, presence, gentle spinal movement, or Spinal Energetics work—signal that it's okay to soften. This is when stored tension begins to unwind.

3. **The spine moves and becomes a pathway for new information**
   As the spine moves more freely and the surrounding tissues soften, communication between brain and body becomes clearer. Instead of reinforcing old protective signals, the system starts sending and receiving more adaptive ones.
4. **Repetition builds a new baseline**
   Healing becomes your natural state, not through a single release, but through repeated experiences of coming out of protection, returning to regulation, and allowing movement instead of holding. Over time, the nervous system learns: *I don't need to brace by default anymore.*
5. **The system reorganizes, not just releases**
   You're now teaching the body a new way to be. One that is responsive instead of reactive, fluid instead of rigid and grounded instead of guarded. Healing stops being something you *do* and becomes something the body naturally returns to. In that state, tension can still arise but it doesn't get stuck. The system knows how to process it, move it, and let it go.

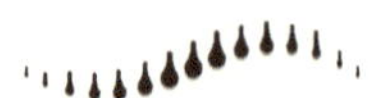

That's what "rewiring" really is: not forcing change but creating the conditions where the body chooses a different pattern, again and again, until that pattern becomes its new normal.

This is how people stay out of chronic pain and regain their health and mobility.

Many modern modalities or personal development courses focus on creating powerful shifts in a person's state through temporary highs of peak emotion, motivation, or mindset tactics. These can be profound in the moment, but they often plateau when a person returns to their everyday environment. This happens because the external environment remains unchanged, and over time, it reshapes the individual back into familiar patterns. As contemplative author Alexander den Heijer points out, "When a flower doesn't bloom, you fix the environment in which it grows, not the flower."

If your environment remains unchanged, patterns can repeat from the external influence it is surrounded by. Rather than relying on external change, Spinal Energetics sees the field as one whole and works to transform the internal landscape so that the external world begins to reflect that change. This makes the transformation more sustainable and less likely to fade over time, as it originates from within rather than being imposed on from outside requirements.

A common challenge in personal development is maintaining connection to moments of clarity or expansion—such as those experienced in retreats, travel, or deeply immersive environments. In these settings, people often feel connected to something greater, to nature, or to a deeper sense of self. The difficulty lies in returning home and sustaining that connection.

Spinal Energetics addresses this by helping individuals cultivate that sense of connection internally, so that their everyday environment becomes meaningful and aligned rather than dependent on external circumstances. At the same time, it does not encourage passive acceptance. There must still be enough internal tension—an awareness of misalignment—to drive meaningful change.

This work is not a cure-all. No modality can resolve every problem or eliminate all struggles. Instead, it offers a different way of seeing oneself and the world. It invites individuals to perceive life through their own authentic perspective, rather than through inherited beliefs or external expectations.

Unlike approaches that rely heavily on discipline or repetition, Spinal Energetics tends to ignite something intrinsic. It becomes less about completing a task and more about **maintaining a relationship with oneself.**

The process doesn't encourage dependence on the modality but focuses on teaching others how to access and trust what already exists within them. In this sense, it teaches people how to "fish" rather than "fishing" for them via temporary solutions.

Sessions evolve into opportunities to reconnect with something already known but not always consciously accessed. The work is both structured and experiential. Participants are required to engage intellectually and emotionally while simultaneously undergoing their own internal process. This creates a dynamic where they are learning and receiving at the same time. It bridges analytical understanding with embodied experience, or in other words, a meeting point between Western structure and Eastern philosophy.

Recognizing What You're Holding

Every pattern in the body was created for a reason. It is the result of your innate intelligence responding to an experience, a moment, or an environment where something was required—protection, control, stability, or adaptation.

So the question isn't, *How do I get rid of this?* But, *Why is this here and is it still needed?*

Not all patterns are meant to be released. Some are supportive, others are stabilizing, and some are part of your natural way of being.

The spine itself reflects this truth. It is not rigid, nor is it loose and unstable. It is strong, adaptable, and responsive. It is designed to move with life, not against it. Healing, then, is not about eliminating all tension but restoring flexible alignment within the system. In Spinal Energetics, we are reading the field and sensing where energy is flowing, where it is held, and where it has become stuck in time. This reveals patterns: outdated ones as well as supportive ones.

An outdated pattern is one where the body is still organizing itself around a past experience, even though the present moment no longer requires that level of protection. Outdated patterns often feel:

- Rigid and repetitive

- Disconnected from what is happening now
- Rooted in unresolved emotional, mental, or energetic layers
- Depleting to the system rather than supportive

They are not "wrong"—they are simply no longer relevant to your current reality.

A supportive pattern, on the other hand, is alive. It adapts, responds, and moves with you. Supportive patterns often feel:

- Flexible and responsive
- Connected to the present moment
- Grounding and stabilizing
- Aligned with what your system actually needs now

They are expressions of a nervous system that feels safe enough to be in flow.

Three Pillars of Somatic Reconnection

The same intelligence that created the pattern is the intelligence that knows how to release it. When you bring awareness to a pattern, when you feel it without judgment, you are essentially communicating with that intelligence.

You are saying: *I see you. I understand why you're here. But we are safe now.*

And when the system truly feels that, it shifts to safety. The field reorganizes, the nervous system softens, and the spine begins to move differently.

1. Mindful Awareness

The first step in healing is *awareness.*

Before anything can change, it must first be noticed. Your posture is never random. The way you sit, stand, and move is shaped by years of physical, emotional and psychological experiences. The tightness in your shoulders, the guarding in your chest, the rigidity in your lower back are not just mechanical issues; they are patterns. And patterns are observable.

Bring your attention into your body. Start by noticing:

- Where do you hold tension without realizing it?
- Does your body brace in certain situations?
- Do your shoulders lift when you feel overwhelmed?
- Does your breath shorten when you feel unsafe?

These are subtle but powerful cues. Don't judge or try to fix it, just simply witness. The moment you observe a pattern, you are no longer fully inside it and therefore you can simply see it for what it is.

Notice your breath. Notice where your body feels open and where it feels restricted.

Notice without needing to change anything. Awareness creates space. And space is where healing and insight occurs. Once you begin to observe, the next question naturally arises: *What am I holding onto, and does it still belong to me?*

The body is incredibly intelligent. It creates tension and protective strategies for a reason. At some point in your life, that pattern was necessary. It helped you cope, adapt or survive. But the body does not automatically update itself. It will continue running the same pattern long after the original moment until you bring awareness to it. This is why healing is not about removing tension blindly but understanding it.

Ask yourself:

- *Is this tension protecting me from something that is still present?*
- *Is it protecting me from something that is already over?*

There is a difference between present danger and past memory. And the body often cannot tell the difference until you help it.

2. Gentle Movement

The body does not need to be forced into alignment—it needs safety and encouragement to move. Slow, intuitive movement allows the nervous system to feel safe enough to release tension. This could be stretching, yoga, swimming, dancing, walking, or simply allowing your body to move in ways that feel natural rather than prescribed. When movement is guided by awareness, it becomes a somatic conversation rather than a correction. We are born to move, and our body feels right when we do.

3. Intentional Release

Release is what happens once the body feels safe. Sometimes this presents as a deep breath, a subtle shift in posture or an energy boost. It can also feel like freedom is emerging, a flexibility towards life, an emotional change, a burden lifted off your shoulders.

The intention is to not force the body into letting go but showing it that it no longer needs to hold on.

The Return to Flow

When awareness, movement, and intention come together, something begins to shift. The body relaxes and the breath deepens. The spine begins to flex and stabilize more freely. Not because you forced it, but because you stopped interfering with it. Healing is a return. A return to flow, to safety. A return to yourself. And perhaps most importantly, remembering that your body has known how to heal all along.

Applying the Practices to Spinal Archetypes

The practices of mindful awareness, gentle movement, and intentional release are not one-size-fits-all. They become powerful when they are directed toward the specific patterns your body is expressing. The Spinal Archetypes we explored in chapter 5 show the patterns embedded in our bodies. Each holds a different story, so each requires a slightly different doorway back to balance.

When you relate the practices to the archetypes, healing becomes more precise because you're communicating directly with the pattern your body is holding. You are saying:

- *I see why you're here.*
- *I understand what you were protecting.*
- *And I'm safe enough now to begin letting go.*

Real change happens through an intimate, listening relationship. It bridges:

1. The **physical body** (spine, fascia, movement)
2. The **nervous system** (regulation, safety, adaptation)
3. The **energetic and perceptual layers** (patterns, awareness, stored experiences)

Rather than separating these domains, they recognize that each one influences the others continuously. Integrating mind, body, and spirit doesn't mean abandoning science—it means expanding it. It means being open to multiple layers of understanding, while still grounding care in safety, evidence, and critical thinking.

Healing Patterns of the Lower Back (Lumbar)—Safety and Support

The lower back is the foundation of your spine, both structurally and energetically. It is where your sense of safety, stability, and trust in the world is anchored. When this area is in balance, there is a quiet sense of being held: by the ground beneath you, by life itself, and by your own internal strength. When it is not, the body organizes itself into patterns of either over-holding or under-supporting.

- The Lone Wolf archetype holds tension through over-responsibility and self-reliance. The body braces, flattening the natural curve, as if preparing to carry everything alone.
- The Dependent archetype holds tension through a lack

of internal grounding and over-reliance on others. The lower back collapses into an exaggerated curve, searching for support.

Both patterns are asking the same important questions: *Am I safe? And can I trust support?*

Mindful Awareness for the Lower Back

Healing the lumbar spine begins with bringing awareness to your relationship with support—not just physically, but emotionally and energetically. Notice how you move through life:

- Do you feel like everything rests on your shoulders?
- Do you struggle to ask for help, even when you need it?
- Or do you feel unsteady, like you can't quite hold yourself up without reassurance from others?
- Do you describe life such as "back-breaking" or "carrying a heavy load"?

Bring awareness into your body and place attention on your lower back. Feel the weight of your body meeting the ground beneath you.

Ask yourself, gently: *Am I supported right now?*

Feel the question rather than think about it. Often, the body is safer than the mind believes. And sometimes simply recognizing present-moment support begins to soften years of unconscious holding. Support can take many forms: financial, emotional, practical, relational and physical.

You can also write what arises for you.

Gentle Movement for the Lower Back

The lumbar spine does not respond well to force or overriding it—it responds to safety. Grounded, rhythmic movement helps the nervous system shift out of protection and into trust.

This can look like:

- Slow walking, feeling each step connect you to the ground
- Gentle swaying of the hips, allowing the pelvis to move freely
- Pelvic tilts or circles that reintroduce fluidity into the lower spine
- Yoga postures that emphasize grounding—where the body is supported, not strained

The intention is not to stretch or fix the lower back, but to **remind it that it is supported**.

As movement becomes slower and more conscious, the body begins to reorganize.

The breath drops deeper, and the muscles ease their tension. The lumbar spine starts to find its natural curve again because it feels safe enough to return.

Intentional Release for the Lower Back

Release in the lower back is connected to trust. This is not just a physical letting go—it is a nervous system shift.

For the Lone Wolf, release looks like softening the grip of control. It may feel unfamiliar to:

- Let someone help you
- Lean into support
- Not carry everything alone

But each time you allow support, whether it's resting your body, receiving help, or even emotionally opening, you send a new signal to the spine: *You don't have to hold this by yourself anymore.*

For the Dependent, release looks like reclaiming internal stability. It is the subtle but powerful shift of:

- Feeling your feet on the ground
- Engaging your own strength
- Trusting your ability to hold yourself

Rather than reaching outward for constant reassurance, the body begins to root inward.

You begin to feel: *I can support myself.*

Healing Patterns of the Upper Back (Thoracic)—Heart and Protection

The upper back is the home of the heart space. It is where we hold our capacity to give and receive love, to feel connection, and to remain open in the presence of life. When this area is balanced, there is a natural openness through the chest—an ease in breathing, in relating, and in being seen. When it is not, the body organizes itself around protection.

- The Hunch archetype protects the heart by closing it. The shoulders round forward, the chest collapses, and the body subtly withdraws from the world.
- The Shield archetype protects by doing the opposite—it becomes rigid, armored, and disconnected from feeling. The chest may appear open structurally, but there is a lack of true emotional availability behind it.

Both are intelligent strategies and attempts to avoid pain.

And both are asking the same question: *Is it safe for me to feel and be open?*

Mindful Awareness for the Upper Back

Healing the thoracic spine begins with awareness of how you protect your heart. Start by noticing your posture in everyday moments:

- Do your shoulders roll forward when you feel uncomfortable or exposed?
- Do you subtly collapse inward in certain conversations or environments?
- Or do you hold yourself upright and composed, but feel emotionally distant or guarded beneath the surface?

Bring your awareness to your chest and upper back. Notice the space across your collarbones. Notice the tone of the muscles between your shoulder blades. Notice your breath—does it reach into the ribcage or stay shallow?

Then ask yourself, gently: *What am I protecting my heart from?*

Often people try to protect their heart from further pain: heartbreak, rejection, isolation, hurt.

Just sense and feel what comes up. Sometimes the answer will be clear. Other times it will simply be a feeling of tightness, heaviness, or numbness. That is normal and natural. Awareness begins to see the protection without forcing it.

You can also write what arises for you.

....

....

....

....

....

....

....

....

....

....

....

....

Gentle Movement for the Upper Back

The thoracic spine responds to softness in a unique way. It doesn't require "standing up straight" or pulling your shoulders back into an artificial posture. That often reinforces the Shield.

Instead, think of movement as an invitation.

- Small, slow expansions through the chest
- Gentle shoulder rolls that release accumulated tension
- Subtle movements that allow the ribcage to widen and soften
- Breathing practices that expand the back of the heart, not just the front

The key is that the movement feels safe.

For the Hunch, movement is about *gradual opening*, like letting light in through a door that has been closed for a long time. For the Shield, movement is about *reintroducing fluidity*—allowing rigidity to soften without losing a sense of safety.

Even something as simple as placing a hand on your chest and breathing into that space can begin to restore connection. Because the thoracic spine is not just moved by muscles; it is deeply influenced by the breath and the invitation to feel love.

Intentional Release for the Upper Back

Release in the upper back is about allowing the heart to feel again, but only at a pace the nervous system can handle.

For the Hunch, release does not mean suddenly opening fully. That can feel overwhelming or unsafe. Instead, it is about allowing small moments of openness:

- Letting your chest soften slightly
- Allowing yourself to be seen in safe environments
- Receiving connection without immediately withdrawing

Each small opening sends a message to the body: *It is safe to come out of protection.*

For the Shield, release looks different. It is less about opening up, and more about *feeling more*. This may begin with:

- Noticing subtle emotions in the body
- Allowing sensation without immediately analyzing or shutting it down

- Letting the breath deepen into areas that feel numb or distant

The Shield often fears being overwhelmed by emotion. So the work is to show the body that feeling can happen in a controlled, safe and grounded way.

As the thoracic patterns begin, the heart space opens and feels less need to hide and armor itself. It increases its capacity to experience life as it is, without needing to constantly protect against it. This is the balance of the upper back: to be open and responsive and safe enough to feel without being fully exposed or closed. And from this place, connection with yourself naturally occurs.

Healing Patterns for the Neck (Cervical)—Mind, Expression and Control

The neck is the bridge between the head and the body—between thinking and feeling, control and surrender, expression and suppression. It is where your internal world meets your external voice. When this area is balanced, there is fluid communication between mind and body. Thoughts are integrated with feeling. Expression is clear, grounded, and authentic. When it is not, the system becomes divided.

- The Overachiever archetype holds tension through constant mental activity, control, and striving. The head leads; the body follows.
- The Metamorphosis archetype holds tension through suppressed truth or the friction of becoming. There is

something within that wants to be expressed but hasn't yet found a safe way to emerge.

Both patterns reflect a disconnect, either from the body below or from the truth within. And both are asking the same question: *Is it safe for me to let go and fully express myself?*

Mindful Awareness for the Neck

Healing the cervical spine begins with noticing where your attention lives. For many people, it is almost entirely in the head.

Observe your internal state:

- Are you constantly thinking, planning, analyzing?
- Do you find it difficult to switch off or be still?
- Do you feel disconnected from your body, as if you're "living upstairs"?

Or on the other side:

- Do you feel like there are things you want to say but don't?
- Do you hold back your truth to avoid conflict or discomfort?
- Do you feel tension in your throat when you try to express yourself?

Bring awareness to your neck. Notice the muscles at the base of your skull. Notice the front of your throat: Is there any tightness, restriction, or subtle holding?

Then ask yourself: *Am I thinking instead of feeling? Is there something I'm not expressing?*

Let the question land in the body, not just the mind. Because often, the neck tightens when the mind overrides the body or when the body holds back what needs to be said. Expression issues can be difficulty in communicating something important, a lack of expression, needing to remain silent about something you're conflicted about, or your expression and voice being suppressed.

You can also write what arises for you.

....

....

....

....

....

....

....

....

....

....

....

....

Gentle Movement for the Neck

The cervical spine thrives on slow, conscious, connected movement. It's not about stretching to extremes, but engaging in awareness-led motion. This can look like:

- Slow rotations of the head, noticing where movement feels restricted
- Gentle nodding or tilting, reconnecting the head to the spine
- Allowing the neck to move in a way that feels intuitive rather than prescribed

Gentle movement is felt, not stretched or performed.

For the Overachiever, movement is about *coming down out of the head* by letting the neck soften so the body can rejoin the experience. For the Metamorphosis, movement is about *creating space* by loosening the areas where expression has been held or restricted.

Even subtle awareness, like feeling the weight of your head resting on your spine, can begin to shift the pattern. Because the neck is not just holding tension; it is holding direction, control, and unspoken truth.

Intentional Release for the Neck

Release in the cervical spine is deeply connected to surrender and expression.

For the Overachiever, release means letting go of control, if only for a moment. This might look like:

- Allowing stillness without needing to fill it
- Letting the mind slow down, even briefly
- Trusting that you don't need to think your way through everything

The tension in the neck softens when the system realizes: *I don't have to hold everything together through effort.*

For the Metamorphosis, release is about gradual expression. This could be:

- Speaking something you've been holding back
- Writing without filtering your thoughts

- Acknowledging a truth internally, even if you're not ready to share it yet

The body doesn't need you to have all the answers. It just needs you to stop suppressing what it already knows. Each act of expression sends a signal: *It is safe for my truth to exist.*

You don't have to hold life together through effort. As the cervical patterns begin to unwind, the division between head and body starts to dissolve. The mind quietens and the body becomes more present. Expression feels clearer and easier. There is less gripping at the top of the spine and less need to control every outcome.

There is a more noticeable trust in the natural flow between thinking, feeling and being. This is the natural balance of the neck—not dominated by the mind or silenced from expression. The true nature of the cervical spine is an integrated, fluid, and aligned position where your thoughts, your voice, and your body can finally move together.

Healing Patterns of the Sacrum—Intuition and Inner Trust

The sacrum sits at the base of the spine, and it is your center of gravity, your anchor point, and your connection to both the earth and your inner world. It is often referred to as the "sacred bone," as it is where intuition lives. This is where your body's innate knowing resides before the mind has a chance to interpret or override it.

When this area is balanced, there is a deep sense of inner trust.

You feel grounded, connected, and guided from within. When it is not, the system becomes disconnected or overwhelmed.

- The Pleaser archetype disconnects from inner knowing, constantly orienting outward: seeking validation, approval, and direction from others.
- The Boiling Pot archetype holds tension between anxiety and disconnection, and it is a system caught between the future and the present, unable to settle.

Both patterns lose connection to the same place: *the quiet, grounded voice within.*

And both are asking: *Can I trust myself? Can I feel safe in my own body?*

Mindful Awareness for the Sacrum

Healing the sacrum begins with returning your attention to the base of your body. This is often the area people feel the least connected to, as they are either numb, tense, or simply outside of awareness. Bring your attention to the base of your spine.

Notice:

- The weight of your pelvis
- Your connection to the surface beneath you
- Any sensations: tightness, pressure, or even absence of feeling

Then ask yourself, gently: *What do I actually feel here? Am I listening to myself or to everyone else?*

For the Pleaser, awareness often reveals how quickly attention moves toward others' opinions, expectations and needs.

For the Boiling Pot, awareness may reveal restlessness, agitation, or a subtle sense of unease that is always present beneath the surface. The goal is not to fix what you find but to simply return. The sacrum begins to regulate the moment it is brought back into awareness.

You can also write what arises for you.

....

....

....

....

....

....

....

....

....

....

....

Gentle Movement for the Sacrum

The sacrum responds to fluidity. Unlike areas of the spine that benefit from structure or stability, the sacrum needs to feel movement that is natural, rhythmic and connected.

This can look like:

- Gentle rocking of the pelvis
- Swaying side to side
- Wave-like movements that travel from the base of the spine upward
- Slow, intuitive movements that reconnect the upper and lower body

The intention is not to perform a movement, but to restore communication between the body's foundation and your nervous system.

For the Pleaser, this movement helps bring awareness back inward—away from external orientation and into internal sensation. For the Boiling Pot, it helps discharge excess energy and regulate the nervous system, allowing the body to settle.

As the sacrum begins to move more freely, there is often a sense of softening, not just physically, but emotionally, as this area holds not just tension, suppressed feelings and unprocessed energy.

Intentional Release for the Sacrum

Release in the sacrum is about trust and regulation.

For the Pleaser, release is the act of choosing yourself. This begins in small, quiet ways:

- Making a decision without asking for validation
- Listening to your initial instinct and honoring it
- Noticing when you override your own knowing and choosing differently

Each time you do this, you strengthen the connection back to your inner compass.

You begin to embody this idea: *I can trust what I feel.*

For the Boiling Pot, release is about slowing the system down. The body is often caught in a loop of overactivation, with too much energy moving upward and not enough grounding below.

Release comes through:

- Lengthening the breath, especially the exhale

- Bringing attention back to the present moment
- Feeling the weight of the body supported by the ground

You are not trying to eliminate the energy; you are helping it settle.

And as it does, the nervous system begins to recognize: *I am safe here. I don't need to stay on high alert.*

As sacral patterns begin to unwind, the body reconnects to something deeper than thought. There is less second-guessing, seeking of external validation and underlying anxiety. Instead, there is a sense of being at home within yourself because the sacrum no longer feels disconnected or overwhelmed. It returns to its natural movement of being stable with a fluid foundation.

This is the balance of the sacrum: keeping a rooted and regulated grounding without outsourcing your truth or living in constant tension.

The Future of Medicine

We are standing at the edge of a quiet revolution in medicine. The conventional system, which has long focused on diagnosing, managing, and controlling parts of the body, is now meeting a collective desire for something more.

And while modern medicine has brought extraordinary advancements, it has also left something essential behind: *the part of us that cannot be measured.* The part that intuitively knows something long before symptoms appear. The deeper aspect of us that senses misalignment beyond tools and tests.

Science has come so far, and the future of medicine will not abandon it, but deepen it through expansion.

My vision is that we move beyond what is merely visible and expand into an integrative understanding of the human experience. It's here that energetic medicine will no longer sit on the fringes, but become an essential part of how we understand health, healing, and the body itself.

Spinal Energetics sits at the forefront of this emerging frontier. It is not simply a modality, but a way of relating to life—one that honors the body as intelligent, responsive, and deeply connected. I encourage our Spinal Energetics practitioners to be the future they wish to see. And for me, this evolution is not optional; it's essential. It forms part of my life's purpose and empowers me to offer whatever gifts I have to the collective.

The Future Practitioner

The future practitioner is already here. They are often not seen but they're quietly breaking cycles, walking between worlds, and restoring wholeness to fragmented people, places, and systems.

They understand that healing is not always about removing something, but about restoring the relationship between body and mind, between self and environment, and between awareness and action. They not only read scans and lab results, but they also read the body through energy, presence, perception and attunement.

And of course, technology will advance and AI will play a part in the future of our health; but we, as human beings, are also advanced. Our human superpowers of touch, love, care and intellectual and emotional intelligence make us incredibly unique. Our body's network is alive with nerves, electrical signals and currents that give us somatic awareness and the ability to self-heal and help others.

Somatic awareness is the body's first language of truth, and humans are gifted in this language, but only if we actually listen and observe. The future of medicine will combine advanced technology with advanced humans, and medicine should always restore wholeness and not inflict more harm.

This is where, if handled with care, the future of medicine becomes both more advanced *and* more human. It is about science and sacredness in partnership.

The Future Recipient of Care

Imagine the world of medicine where the individual is no longer a passive recipient of care, but an active and engaged participant in their own healing. Not pushing sole responsibility onto their doctor or allied health practitioner, but instead taking ownership and working in conjunction with those supporting them.

Thinking of medicine through the lens of long-term wellness is new for many. As energetic medicine becomes integrated into traditional medicine, people begin to reconnect with their internal guidance system and they change their relationship to Self in doing so. They learn to recognize early signals. To trust their body. To respond before imbalance becomes illness. This helps the recipient of care take agency and become the instigator of their healing.

And just to be clear, I don't suggest that we fully reject the old systems. Instead, we need to revolutionize them. And how do we do this? Firstly, by widening the scope of what we consider valid, measurable, and real and simultaneously hold space for the unconscious, energetic and spiritual elements too.

It's my hope that the future of medicine will not only treat the body, but also listen to it. And it's also my hope that it will hold our human body as a sacred gift—an intelligent one that is already pointing in the right direction.

And in that paradigm, new possibilities for healing begin to unfold.

"Through Love
all pain will turn
to medicine."

RUMI

Your Personal Pilgrimage

The spine is your bridge to higher awareness of Self. It's the active link between your unconscious and conscious awareness. However, the bridge itself does not do the walking. Everyone must take responsibility for their own movement, choices, and actions. Spinal Energetics makes the crossing clearer and more accessible, but the journey remains personal.

It's also important to recognize that there is a deeper philosophical tension at play: the dance between surrender and action, between destiny and free will. Your growth requires your active engagement and at times, surrender, to something greater. Too much control restricts the process; too much passivity prevents it from unfolding.

Ultimately, Spinal Energetics can be seen as an internal pilgrimage. Like physical pilgrimages taken across sacred landscapes, this work involves moving through layers of self, uncovering meaning, and reconnecting to something deeper. The path exists, but it must be walked.

The spine is the bridge to Self, but walking it takes courage.

It requires courage to look inward. It's often easier to avoid discomfort or remain in familiar terrain and patterns. Yet over time, avoidance accumulates, making the process of facing oneself even more difficult. Engaging with this work consistently allows for ongoing integration, rather than a buildup of unresolved experiences or tensions.

The goal is not to become "fully healed" or perfected. That idea itself can become another form of striving. Instead, the process is one of continual awareness and of being willing to see, to listen, and to evolve.

Rather than "leveling up," it can be understood as a process of *de-layering*. Removing what is not authentic while shedding conditioned identities and returning to the core self. It is less about becoming something new and more about revealing who you truly are.

From this place of alignment, decisions become clearer. You can breathe again and finally act in ways that feel natural to you. Success, then, becomes redefined—not as external achievement or recognition, but as living in accordance with your true self.

And interestingly enough, within this new freedom of Self, external outcomes, such as abundance or recognition, often arise as a byproduct of your new shifts, not as the primary goal. When actions are aligned internally, they tend to resonate outwardly, creating a natural flow rather than a forced pursuit.

At its essence, this work is all about connection—connection to self, to something greater, and to the truth that emerges when we are willing to listen.

It is a great adventure into your own story, the layers that you hold, the experiences you've endured and the evolution of your soul that continues to unfold. It is more of a return than an outward journey.

A remembering of who you were before the world told you who to be.

And somewhere along the way, you realize that you are the hero of this story. But a new type of hero. Not one who conquers through striving or proving, but through the courage to turn inward and keep choosing what is true.

Your spine is your guide. It will always lead you back to alignment. Every movement, every pull, every shift is an invitation to come home. And of course, home is not a destination or place.

It's a return to you.

And your work, and my work too, is to return again and again. Return to the essence of your soul knowing that your spine acts as the living compass to your walk in truth and authenticity.

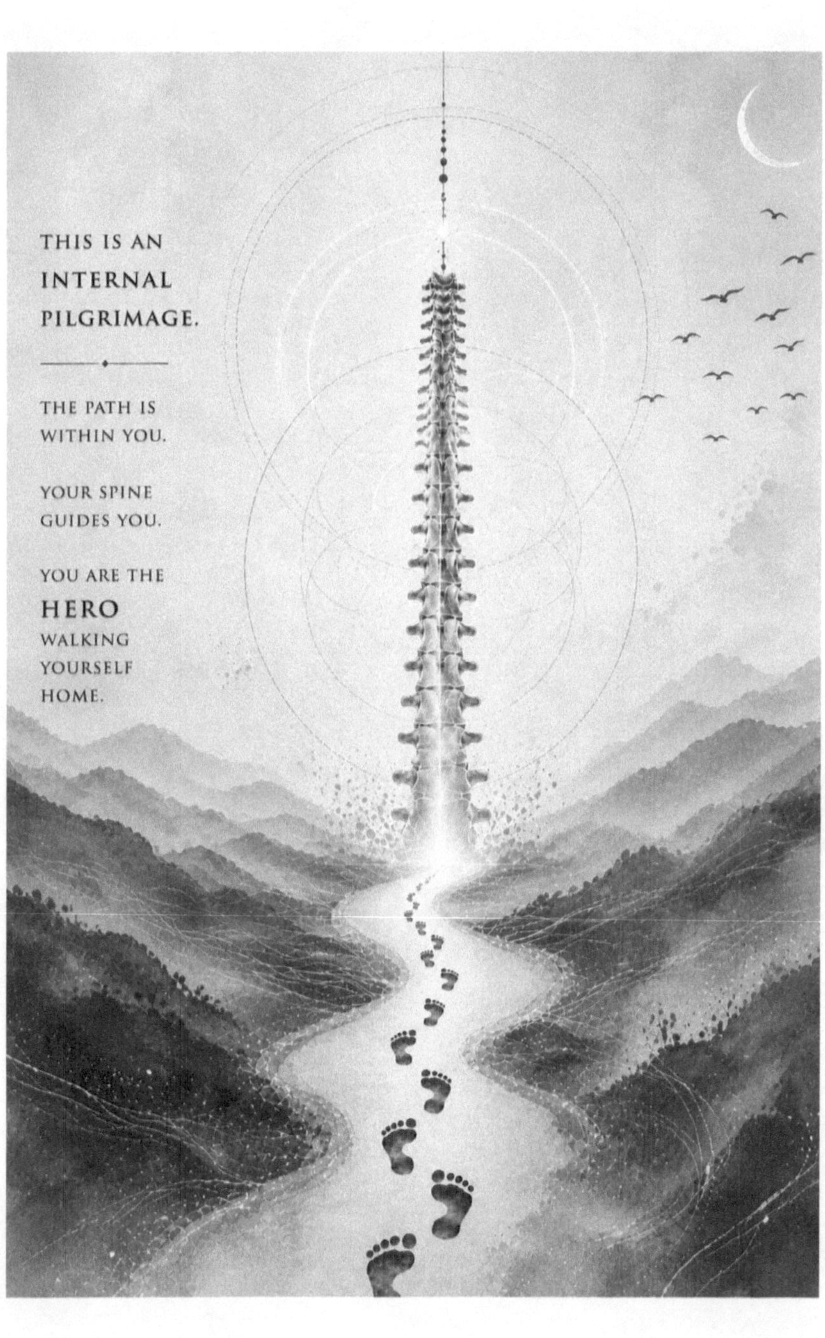
THIS IS AN
INTERNAL
PILGRIMAGE.
THE PATH IS
WITHIN YOU.
YOUR SPINE
GUIDES YOU.
YOU ARE THE
HERO
WALKING
YOURSELF
HOME.

ACKNOWLEDGMENTS

To Barny, whose financial support made studying chiropractic possible when it otherwise would not have been, and whose refusal to let me quit when things got hard shaped everything that followed.

To Dylan, for the depth of our conversations and for being a true soul in this strange and beautiful world.

To Tom, for your encouragement, your uniquely beautiful way of seeing things, and for always allowing me the space to see things my own way.

To Kirsty and Katie, for supporting me both personally and professionally in ways that gave me the freedom and clarity to actually write this book.

To the Spinal Energetics Team and the wider community of practitioners, whose curiosity and hunger for deeper understanding of the spine and its connection to spirituality continually pushed this work further than I imagined it could go.

To chiropractic and to the many teachers, practitioners, and traditions in the healing world who have shaped my understanding and deepened my path.

To my friends and family, who inspire me every day to live a life that is honest and true to who I am. Cooper, Benson and Lou Lou.

And to Nat and Jess for seeing my vision, hearing it fully, and bringing it to life.

About The Author

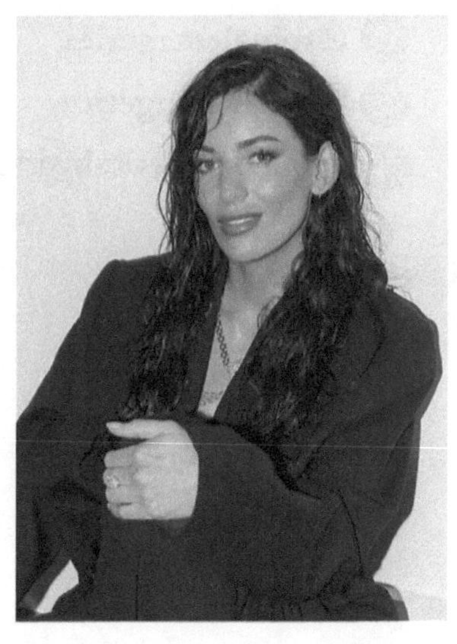

Dr. Sarah Jane is a holistic chiropractor and the founder of Spinal Energetics. She is a renowned teacher and practitioner with an empathetic and kind approach that is anchored by a genuine ability to create rapport and support her clients through her boundless knowledge of the human experience.

Her expertise in philosophy, consciousness, cross-cultural awareness, trauma, energetics, and the human body has earned her thousands of clients from diverse backgrounds, including members of the royal family, therapists, spiritual teachers, musicians, doctors, scientists, athletes, CEOs and celebrities.

Dr. Sarah Jane's process is inclusive, deeply emotive and effective, designed to empower you on your journey through light yet impactful touch and honoring your body's communication.

She brings a multifaceted, energetic, and efficient approach through the latest techniques and by working within an evidence-based framework. She shares her wisdom through various speaking engagements, workshops, training, and private and group sessions.

spinalenergetics.com
drsarahjanechiro.com.au
@spinalenergetics
@spinalenergetics
spinalenergeticsbydrsarahjane

Stay Connected

Learn more about Spinal Energetics and stay connected to our community and events.

Spinal Energetics

spinalenergetics.com

Self Practice

Find a Practitioner

Become a Practitioner

Ebook - The Body's Hidden Messages

AUDIOBOOK

Great news! *Your Spine Holds The Answer* is also available in audio format. Jump onto your favourite audiobook platform now and check it out.

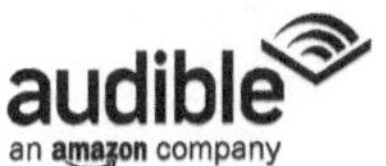

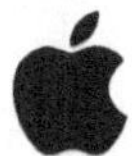

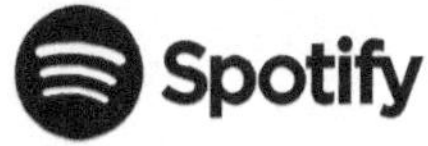

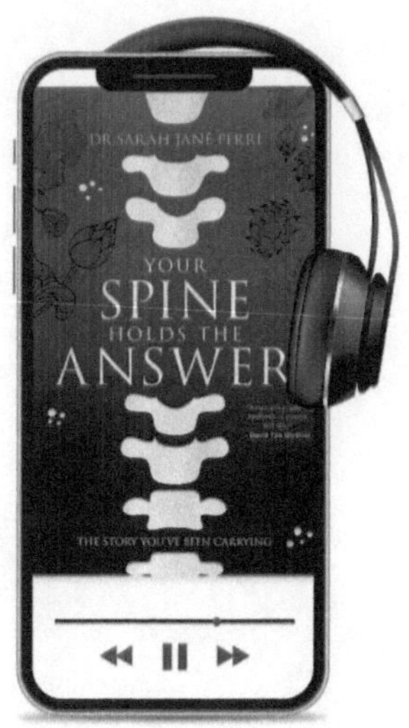

ENDNOTES

1 Jung, C. G. 1998. *Jung's Seminar on Nietzsche's Zarathustra.* Edited by James L. Jarrett. Abridged ed. Princeton, NJ: Princeton University Press.

2 Pauli W. The influence of archetypal ideas on the scientific theories of Kepler. The Interpretation of nature and the psyche, 1955, Routledge & Kegan Paul. London.

3 Di Carlo, F., Vicinelli, M. C., Pettorruso, M., De Risio, L., Migliara, G., Baccolini, V., Trioni, J., Grant, J. E., Dell'Osso, B., & Martinotti, G. (2024). Connected minds in disconnected bodies: Exploring the role of interoceptive sensibility and alexithymia in problematic use of the internet. *Comprehensive psychiatry*, *129*, 152446.

4 Marais, E. N. (1969). *The Soul of the Ape.* Atheneum.

5 Close, Frank. *The Void. Oxford: Oxford University Press*, 2007; Halliday, David, Robert Resnick, and Jearl Walker. *Fundamentals of Physics*. 10th ed. Hoboken, NJ: Wiley, 2013.

6 Ibid.

7 Ibid.

8 Galvani, Luigi. De viribus electricitatis in motu musculari [Commentary on the Effect of Electricity on Muscular Motion]. Bologna: Ex Typographia Instituti Scientiarum, 1791; Piccolino, Marco. "Animal Electricity and the Birth of Electrophysiology: The Legacy of Luigi Galvani." Brain Research Bulletin 46, no. 5 (1998): 381–407.

9 Kane, Suzanne Amador, and Boris A. Gelman. Introduction to Physics in Modern Medicine. 3rd ed. Boca Raton, FL: CRC Press, 2020.

10 Ibid.

11 McCraty, Rollin. *The Energetic Heart: Bioelectromagnetic Interactions Within and Between People*. Boulder Creek, CA: HeartMath Institute, 2004.

12 McCraty, Rollin, Mike Atkinson, and Dana Tomasino. "Touch the Hearts of Men." *The International Journal of Humanities and Peace* 19, no. 1 (2003): 80–84.

13 Burr, Harold Saxton. Blueprint for Immortality: The Electric Patterns of Life. London: Neville Spearman, 1972.

14 Burr, H. S., and F. S. C. Northrop. "The Electro-Dynamic Theory of Life." The Quarterly Review of Biology 10, no. 3 (September 1935): 322–333.

15 Burr, Harold S., George M. Smith, and Leone C. Strong. 1938. "Bio-Electric Properties of Cancer-Resistant and Cancer-Susceptible Mice." *The American Journal of Cancer* 32 (2): 240–48.

16 Langevin, H. M., & Yandow, J. A. (2002). Relationship of acupuncture points and meridians to connective tissue planes. *The Anatomical Record, 15*;269(6):257-65. https://doi.org/10.1002/ar.10185.

17 Halliday, David, Robert Resnick, and Jearl Walker. *Fundamentals of Physics*. 10th ed. Hoboken, NJ: John Wiley & Sons, 2013.

18 Zimmerman, John. "New Technologies Detect Effects of Healing Hands." Brain/Mind Bulletin 10, no. 16 (1985): 3.

19 Clayton, M. (2012). What is entrainment? Definition and applications in musical research. Empirical Musicology Review, 7(1-2), 49-56. https://kb.osu.edu/dspace/bitstream/handle/1811/52979/EMR000137a-Clayton.pdf

20 Barbaresi, Marco et al. "Physiological Entrainment: A Key Mind-Body Mechanism for Cognitive, Motor and Affective Functioning, and Well-Being." *Brain sciences, 15*. https://doi.org/10.3390/brainsci15010003.

21 Gordon, E.M., Chauvin, R.J., Van, A.N. et al. A somato-cognitive action network alternates with effector regions in motor cortex. Nature 617, 351–359 (2023). https://doi.org/10.1038/s41586-023-05964-2

22 Vanutelli, Maria Elide et al. "Editorial: Moving the mind, thinking the body: new insights on the mind–body connection from the neuroscience of movement, sports, arts, yoga, and meditation." *Frontiers in human neuroscience* vol. 18 1376909. 7 Feb. 2024, doi:10.3389/fnhum.2024.1376909

23 Querdasi, Francesca R, and Bridget L Callaghan. "A Translational Approach to the Mind-Brain-Body Connection." *Translational issues in psychological science* vol. 9,2 (2023): 103-106. doi:10.1037/tps0000374

24 Nelson CA, Scott RD, Bhutta ZA, Harris NB, Danese A, & Samara M (2020). Adversity in childhood is linked to mental and physical health throughout life. BMJ, 371, Article m3048. 10.1136/BMJ.M3048.

25 Sartorious N (2013). Comorbidity of mental and physical diseases: A main challenge for medicine of the 21st century. Shanghai Archives of Psychiatry, 25(2), 68–69. 10.3969/j.issn.1002-0829.2013.02.002.

26 Goldberg, Daniel S, and Summer J McGee. "Pain as a global public health priority." *BMC public health* vol. 11 770. 6 Oct. 2011, doi:10.1186/1471-2458-11-770.

27 Chronic Pain Australia. 2024 National Pain Report: The Social and Economic Cost of Chronic Pain. Sydney: Chronic Pain Australia, 2024.

28 Chronic Pain Australia. 2024 National Pain Report: The Social and Economic Cost of Chronic Pain. Sydney: Chronic Pain Australia, 2024.

29 Allis, C. David, Thomas Jenuwein, and Danny Reinberg. 2007. *Epigenetics*. Cold Spring Harbor, NY: Cold Spring Harbor Laboratory Press.

30 Lipton, Bruce H. 2005. *The Biology of Belief: Unleashing the Power of Consciousness*, Matter & Miracles. Santa Rosa, CA: Mountain of Love/Elite Books; Lipton, Bruce H., Klaus G. Bensch, and Marvin A. Karasek. 1977. "Microenvironment Controls Morphogenesis in Colonies of Isolated Keratinocytes." *Journal of Investigative Dermatology 68* (5): 272–79.

31 Cole, Steve W., Louise C. Hawkley, Jesusa M. Arevalo, and John T. Cacioppo. 2007. "Social Regulation of Gene Expression in Human Leukocytes." *Genome Biology 8* (9): R189.

32 Sapolsky, Robert M. 2004. *Why Zebras Don't Get Ulcers: The Acclaimed Guide to Stress, Stress-Related Diseases, and Coping*. 3rd ed. New York: Henry Holt and Company.

33 Segerstrom, Suzanne C., and Gregory E. Miller. 2004. "Psychological Stress and the Human Immune System: A Meta-Analytic Study of 30 Years of Inquiry." *Psychological Bulletin 130* (4): 601–30.

34 Cohen, Sheldon, Denise Janicki-Deverts, William J. Doyle, Gregory E. Miller, Ellen Frank, Bruce S. Rabin, and Ronald B. Turner. 2012. "Chronic Stress, Glucocorticoid Receptor Resistance, Inflammation, and Disease Risk." *Proceedings of the National Academy of Sciences 109* (16): 5995–99.

35 Cohen S. (1995). Psychological stress and susceptibility to upper respiratory infections. *American journal of respiratory and critical*

care medicine, *152*(4 Pt 2), S53–S58. https://doi.org/10.1164/ajrccm/152.4_Pt_2.S53.

36 Sheikh M. A. (2018). Retrospectively reported childhood adversity is associated with asthma and chronic bronchitis, independent of mental health. *Journal of psychosomatic research*, *114*, 50–57. https://doi.org/10.1016/j.jpsychores.2018.09.007.

37 Dispenza, Joe. 2012. *Breaking the Habit of Being Yourself: How to Lose Your Mind and Create a New One*. Carlsbad, CA: Hay House.

38 Rein, Glen, Mike Atkinson, and Rollin McCraty. "The Physiological and Psychological Effects of Compassion and Anger." Journal of Advancement in Medicine 8, no. 2 (1995): 87–105; Dispenza, Joe. *You Are the Placebo: Making Your Mind Matter*. Carlsbad, CA: Hay House, 2014.

39 Dispenza, Joe. 2017. *Becoming Supernatural: How Common People Are Doing the Uncommon*. Carlsbad, CA: Hay House.

40 Van der Kolk, Bessel A. 2014. The Body Keeps the Score: Brain, Mind, and Body in the Healing of Trauma. New York: Viking.

41 Rauch, Scott L., Bessel A. van der Kolk, Robert E. Fisler, Nathaniel M. Alpert, Scott P. Orr, Cary R. Savage, Bruce Fischman, Michael A. Jenike, and Roger K. Pitman. 1996. "A Symptom Provocation Study of Posttraumatic Stress Disorder Using Positron Emission Tomography and Script-Driven Imagery." Archives of General Psychiatry 53 (5): 380–87.

42 Van der Kolk, Bessel A. 2014. The Body Keeps the Score: Brain, Mind, and Body in the Healing of Trauma. New York: Viking.

43 Maté, Gabor. 2003. *When the Body Says No: The Cost of Hidden Stress*. Toronto: Knopf Canada.

44 Temoshok, Lydia. 1987. "Personality, Coping Style, Emotion and Cancer: Towards an Integrative Model." *Cancer Surveys 6* (3): 545–67.

45 Ibid.

46 Spiegel, David, Joan R. Bloom, H. C. Kraemer, and E. Gottheil. 1989. "Effect of Psychosocial Treatment on Survival of Patients with Metastatic Breast Cancer." The Lancet 334 (8668): 888–91.

47 Maté, Gabor. 2003. *When the Body Says No: The Cost of Hidden Stress*. Toronto: Knopf Canada.

48 Carney, Dana R., Amy J. C. Cuddy, and Andy J. Yap. 2010. "Power Posing: Brief Nonverbal Displays Affect Neuroendocrine Levels and Risk Tolerance." *Psychological Science* 21 (10): 1363–68. https://doi.org/10.1177/0956797610383437.

49 Kross, Ethan, Marc G. Berman, Walter Mischel, Edward E. Smith, and Tor D. Wager. 2011. "Social Rejection Shares Somatosensory Representations with Physical Pain." Proceedings of the National Academy of Sciences 108 (15): 6270–75; Eisenberger NI (2012) "The neural bases of social pain," Psychosomatic Medicine, 74(2):126–135, doi:10.1097/psy.0b013e3182464dd1.

50 McEwen, Bruce S. "Neurobiological and Systemic Effects of Chronic Stress." *Chronic stress (Thousand Oaks, Calif.)* vol. 1 (2017): 2470547017692328. doi:10.1177/2470547017692328.

51 Nishitani, S., Fujisawa, T.X., Takiguchi, S. *et al.* Multi-epigenome-wide analyses and meta-analysis of child maltreatment in judicial autopsies and intervened children and adolescents. *Mol Psychiatry* 31, 1253–1264 (2026). https://doi.org/10.1038/s41380-025-03236-1.

52 Kellermann N. P. (2001). Transmission of Holocaust trauma--an integrative view. *Psychiatry*, *64*(3), 256–267. https://doi.org/10.1521/psyc.64.3.256.18464.

53 Van der Kolk, Bessell. A. (2014). *The body keeps the score: Brain, mind, and body in the healing of trauma.* Viking.

54 Weiss, Robert S. 1973. *Loneliness: The Experience of Emotional and Social Isolation.* MIT Press.

55 Schwartz, Barry. 2004. *The Paradox of Choice: Why More Is Less.* New York: Ecco.

56 Ware, Bronnie. 2012. *The Top Five Regrets of the Dying: A Life Transformed by the Dearly Departing.* Carlsbad, CA: Hay House.

www.ingramcontent.com/pod-product-compliance
Lightning Source LLC
Chambersburg PA
CBHW030343280726
48882CB00025B/359

9781764372329